This Guide will teach you to ignore the voices.

Remember: even if you cannot stop the voices, the voices cannot stop you to live a normal life.

If you believe in things which other people consider strange, try to keep your strange believes for yourself. Everybody has to make the selection of what can be told to other people and what must be private. Believe me, many people have strange believes. Even much stranger than yours. And they are not considered to be sick. Why? Because they keep their strange believes for themselves. That is the secret.

***

Afternoon

* Think of three different words, any words which just come to your mind at the moment and make a simple story using these 3 words. Repeat 3 times.

* Try to concentrate on an object close to you, any object. What do you feel when looking at the object? What thoughts come to your mind when looking at the object?

* Dinner and half an hour break (you can sleep).

* Nice talk (no complaints) 15 min. When nobody to talk with, phone or internet conversation oral or written.

* Walk 20 min.

* If you hear voices which are not heard by other people, ask yourself if it is possible to ignore them.

Yes

Great! In such a case continue ignoring them.

No

You have to learn to ignore the voices.

This Guide will teach you to ignore the voices.

Remember: even if you cannot stop the voices, the voices cannot stop you to live a normal life.

If you believe in things which other people consider strange, try to keep your strange believes for yourself. Everybody has to make the selection of what can be told to other people and what must be private. Believe me, many people have strange believes. Even much stranger than yours. And they are not considered to be sick. Why? Because they keep their strange believes for themselves. That is the secret.

***

Can one live, work and be happy with schizophrenia in a normal way, the way people without schizophrenia can? Yes! You can live a normal life with schizophrenia. In order to do so there are only 3 steps to do.

First, you should forget schizophrenia is a disease, so consequently you are not sick! Of course, you experience some psyche disturbances, but there is no human being on Earth with no disturbance. The number of such disturbances is limitless. But people suffering other disturbances are not considered as sick! Why? It is the question of the history. Some disturbances have become in the 20th century more popularized than others. Since psychiatrists are doctors of medecine they used to call these disturbances „diseases", what is quite easy to understand. But people suffer from limitless number of another different psyche disturbances, which have not become as popular in the 20th century as schizophrenia, depression or anxiety. Believe me, there is no man on Earth without this or that disturbance. Most of us is not treated by psychiatrists because they deal only with the 3 most popular disturbances: schizophrenia, depression, anxiety. But it does not mean that these are the only disturbances and that these are „diseases". The truth is that there are no diseases in the psychiatry. There are only disturbances.

Second, as the system of the medical care (psychiatrists, hospitals, pharma industry, law, etc) makes permanently sick person out of you, with a label of schizophrenia disease, you have to came back to normal life on your own. But not alone!

Third, you have to be accompanied in your come back to normal life by somobody close to you: a member of your family, friend, anyone you can rely on and someone with no official psychiatric label. It is hard to find such a person, even in the family, because most of the people accept without reflection what doctors (psychiatrists) tell them. They belive in what doctors say, not you. But this book can help you to explain it to your family and friends that you are not sick and your desire to live a normal life is fully justified. Remember to show to the people this book. It will open your way to normal life.

In this Guide you will find out how you should proceed step by step, day after day, in order to get rid of this false label of schizophrenia, that you are sick. And you will find out how you can overcome your schizophrenic disturbance in order to live a full and normal live.

Follow this Guide step by step and after 3 months you can be sure to be a normal person with your disturbance under control. It means in 3 month you will be no schizophrenic person, but a normal one.

Month one

Week One

Day 1

Morning

* Say STOP when the voices you hear in your head become too loud to hear your own thoughts.

* If above does not help to stop the voices, just turn your attention away from the voices. The best way to turn your attention away from the voices in your head is by doing one of your favorite occupations. Do not be ashamed of any occupation to turn your attention away from the voices in your head. ALWAYS be busy with your favorite occupation when unsupportable voices come to your head.

* Be careful to keep for yourself these of your believes which are found to be strange by the people.

* CONTROL what you say. Say only things which are not strange for the people. You surely already know which of your believes are found to be strange by the people.

* If you do not know yet which of your believes are found to be strange by the people, OBSERVE how

people react on what you say. If you see that people are ALERTED by your believes, it means your believes are strange. From now on AVOID presenting such believes.

* Think of three different words, any words which just come to your mind at the moment and make a simple story using these 3 words. Repeat 3 times.

* Try to concentrate on an object close to you, any object. What do you feel when looking at the object? What thoughts come to your mind when looking at the object?

* Small physical excercise (10 min)

* Small breakfast.

* Nice talk (no complaints, no problematic questions) 10 min. When nobody to talk with, phone or internet conversation oral or written.

* Walk 15 min.

* If you hear voices which are not heard by other people, ask yourself if it is possible to ignore the voices.

Yes

Great! In such a case continue ignoring them.

No

You have to learn to ignore the voices.

Evening

- Think of three different words, any words which just come to your mind at the moment and make a simple story using these 3 words. Repeat 3 times.
  - Try to concentrate on an object close to you, any object. What do you feel when looking at the object? What thoughts come to your mind when looking at the object?
  - Small supper.
  - Nice talk (no complaints) 10 min. When nobody to talk with, phone or internet conversation oral or written.
  - Walk 10 min.
  - If you hear voices which are not heard by other people, ask yourself if it is possible to ignore them.

Yes

Great! In such a case continue ignoring them.

No

You have to learn to ignore the voices.

This Guide will teach you to ignore the voices.

Remember: even if you cannot stop the voices, the voices cannot stop you to live a normal life.

If you believe in things which other people consider strange, try to keep your strange believes for yourself. Everybody has to make the selection of what can be told to other people and what must be private. Believe me, many people have strange believes. Even much stranger than yours. And they are not considered to be sick. Why? Because they keep their strange believes for themselves. That is the secret.

***

Night

Before sleep

- Take a shower (warm water) 1 min.
- Small physical excercise 3 min.

In Bed

- Repeat STOP (10 times if you hear the voices).
- Think of three different words, any words which just come to your mind at the moment and make a simple story using these 3 words. Repeat untill you fall asleep.

If you cannot fall asleep

- Think of three different words, any words which just come to your mind at the moment and make a simple story using these 3 words. Repeat untill you fall asleep.

If above does not help

- Stand up and go to the toilet (when possible with as little light as possible)
- Think of three different words, any words which just come to your mind at the moment and make a simple story using these 3 words. Repeat untill you fall asleep.

If above does not help

- Say STOP untill you fall asleep

If above does not help

- Go to the kitchen and have a very small snack.
- Back to the bed think of three different words, any words which just come to your mind at the moment and make a simple story using these 3 words. Repeat untill you fall asleep.
- If above does not help think of three different words, any words which just come to your mind at the moment and make a simple story using these 3 words. Repeat untill you fall asleep.

***

Day 2

Morning

* Say STOP when the voices you hear in your head become too loud to hear your own thoughts.

* If above does not help to stop the voices, just turn your attention away from the voices. The best way to turn your attention away from the voices in your head is by doing one of your favorite occupations. Do not be ashamed of any occupation to turn your attention away from the voices in your head. ALWAYS be busy with your favorite occupation when unsupportable voices come to your head.

* Be careful to keep for yourself these of your believes which are found to be strange by the people.

* CONTROL what you say. Say only things which are not strange for the people. You surely already know which of your believes are found to be strange by the people.

* If you do not know yet which of your believes are found to be strange by the people, OBSERVE how people react on what you say. If you see that people are ALERTED by your believes, it means your believes are strange. From now on AVOID presenting such believes.

* Think of three different words, any words which just come to your mind at the moment and make a simple story using these 3 words. Repeat 3 times.

* Try to concentrate on an object close to you, any object. What do you feel when looking at the object? What thoughts come to your mind when looking at the object?

* Small physical excercise (10 min)

* Small breakfast.

* Nice talk (no complaints, no problematic questions) 10 min. When nobody to talk with, phone or internet conversation oral or written.

* Walk 15 min.

* If you hear voices which are not heard by other people, ask yourself if it is possible to ignore the voices.

Yes

Great! In such a case continue ignoring them.

No

You have to learn to ignore the voices.

This Guide will teach you to ignore the voices.

Remember: even if you cannot stop the voices, the voices cannot stop you to live a normal life.

If you believe in things which other people consider strange, try to keep your strange believes for yourself. Everybody has to make the selection of what can be told to other people and what must be private. Believe me, many people have strange believes. Even much stranger than yours. And they are not considered to be sick. Why? Because they keep their strange believes for themselves. That is the secret.

***

Afternoon

* Think of three different words, any words which just come to your mind at the moment and make a simple story using these 3 words. Repeat 3 times.

* Try to concentrate on an object close to you, any object. What do you feel when looking at the object? What thoughts come to your mind when looking at the object?

* Dinner and half an hour break (you can sleep).

* Nice talk (no complaints) 15 min. When nobody to talk with, phone or internet conversation oral or written.

* Walk 20 min.

* If you hear voices which are not heard by other people, ask yourself if it is possible to ignore them.

Yes

Great! In such a case continue ignoring them.

No

You have to learn to ignore the voices.

This Guide will teach you to ignore the voices.

Remember: even if you cannot stop the voices, the voices cannot stop you to live a normal life.

If you believe in things which other people consider strange, try to keep your strange believes for yourself. Everybody has to make the selection of what can be told to other people and what must be private. Believe me, many people have strange believes. Even much stranger than yours. And they are not considered to be sick. Why? Because they keep their strange believes for themselves. That is the secret.

***

Evening

- Think of three different words, any words which just come to your mind at the moment and make a simple story using these 3 words. Repeat 3 times.
  - Try to concentrate on an object close to you, any object. What do you feel when looking at the object? What thoughts come to your mind when looking at the object?
  - Small supper.
  - Nice talk (no complaints) 10 min. When nobody to talk with, phone or internet conversation oral or written.
  - Walk 10 min.
  - If you hear voices which are not heard by other people, ask yourself if it is possible to ignore them.

Yes

Great! In such a case continue ignoring them.

No

You have to learn to ignore the voices.

This Guide will teach you to ignore the voices.

Remember: even if you cannot stop the voices, the voices cannot stop you to live a normal life.

If you believe in things which other people consider strange, try to keep your strange believes for yourself. Everybody has to make the selection of what can be told to other people and what must be private. Believe me, many people have strange believes. Even much stranger than yours. And they are not considered to be sick. Why? Because they keep their strange believes for themselves. That is the secret.

***

Night

Before sleep

- Take a shower (warm water) 1 min.
- Small physical excercise 3 min.

In Bed

- Repeat STOP (10 times if you hear the voices.
- Think of three different words, any words which just come to your mind at the moment and make a simple story using these 3 words. Repeat untill you fall asleep.

If you cannot fall asleep

- Think of three different words, any words which just come to your mind at the moment and make a simple story using these 3 words. Repeat untill you fall asleep.

If above does not help

- Stand up and go to the toilet (when possible with as little light as possible)
- Think of three different words, any words which just come to your mind at the moment and make a simple story using these 3 words. Repeat untill you fall asleep.

If above does not help

- Say STOP untill you fall asleep

If above does not help

- Go to the kitchen and have a very small snack.
- Back to the bed think of three different words, any words which just come to your mind at the moment and make a simple story using these 3 words. Repeat untill you fall asleep.
- If above does not help think of three different words, any words which just come to your mind at the moment and make a simple story using these 3 words. Repeat untill you fall asleep.

***

Day 3

Morning

* Say STOP when the voices you hear in your head become too loud to hear your own thoughts.

* If above does not help to stop the voices, just turn your attention away from the voices. The best way to turn your attention away from the voices in your head is by doing one of your favorite occupations. Do not be ashamed of any occupation to turn your attention away from the voices in your head. ALWAYS be busy with your favorite occupation when unsupportable voices come to your head.

* Be careful to keep for yourself these of your believes which are found to be strange by the people.

* CONTROL what you say. Say only things which are not strange for the people. You surely already know which of your believes are found to be strange by the people.

* If you do not know yet which of your believes are found to be strange by the people, OBSERVE how people react on what you say. If you see that people are ALERTED by your believes, it means your believes are strange. From now on AVOID presenting such believes.

* Think of three different words, any words which just come to your mind at the moment and make a simple story using these 3 words. Repeat 3 times.

* Try to concentrate on an object close to you, any object. What do you feel when looking at the object? What thoughts come to your mind when looking at the object?

* Small physical excercise (10 min)

* Small breakfast.

* Nice talk (no complaints, no problematic questions) 10 min. When nobody to talk with, phone or internet conversation oral or written.

* Walk 15 min.

* If you hear voices which are not heard by other people, ask yourself if it is possible to ignore the voices.

Yes

Great! In such a case continue ignoring them.

No

You have to learn to ignore the voices.

This Guide will teach you to ignore the voices.

Remember: even if you cannot stop the voices, the voices cannot stop you to live a normal life.

If you believe in things which other people consider strange, try to keep your strange believes for yourself.

Everybody has to make the selection of what can be told to other people and what must be private. Believe me, many people have strange believes. Even much stranger than yours. And they are not considered to be sick. Why? Because they keep their strange believes for themselves. That is the secret.

***

Afternoon

* Think of three different words, any words which just come to your mind at the moment and make a simple story using these 3 words. Repeat 3 times.

* Try to concentrate on an object close to you, any object. What do you feel when looking at the object? What thoughts come to your mind when looking at the object?

* Dinner and half an hour break (you can sleep).

* Nice talk (no complaints) 15 min. When nobody to talk with, phone or internet conversation oral or written.

* Walk 20 min.

* If you hear voices which are not heard by other people, ask yourself if it is possible to ignore them.

Yes

Great! In such a case continue ignoring them.

No

You have to learn to ignore the voices.

This Guide will teach you to ignore the voices.

Remember: even if you cannot stop the voices, the voices cannot stop you to live a normal life.

If you believe in things which other people consider strange, try to keep your strange believes for yourself. Everybody has to make the selection of what can be told to other people and what must be private. Believe me, many people have strange believes. Even much stranger than yours. And they are not considered to be sick. Why? Because they keep their strange believes for themselves. That is the secret.

***

Evening

- Think of three different words, any words which just come to your mind at the moment and make a simple story using these 3 words. Repeat 3 times.

- Try to concentrate on an object close to you, any object. What do you feel when looking at the object? What thoughts come to your mind when looking at the object?
- Small supper.
- Nice talk (no complaints) 10 min. When nobody to talk with, phone or internet conversation oral or written.
- Walk 10 min.
- If you hear voices which are not heard by other people, ask yourself if it is possible to ignore them.

Yes

Great! In such a case continue ignoring them.

No

You have to learn to ignore the voices.

This Guide will teach you to ignore the voices.

Remember: even if you cannot stop the voices, the voices cannot stop you to live a normal life.

If you believe in things which other people consider strange, try to keep your strange believes for yourself. Everybody has to make the selection of what can be told to other people and what must be private. Believe me, many people have strange believes. Even much stranger than yours. And they are not considered to be sick. Why? Because they keep their strange believes for themselves. That is the secret.

***

Night

Before sleep

- Take a shower (warm water) 1 min.
- Small physical excercise 3 min.

In Bed

- Repeat STOP (10 times if you hear the voices.
- Think of three different words, any words which just come to your mind at the moment and make a simple story using these 3 words. Repeat untill you fall asleep.

If you cannot fall asleep

- Think of three different words, any words which just come to your mind at the moment and make a simple story using these 3 words. Repeat untill you fall asleep.

If above does not help

- Stand up and go to the toilet (when possible with as little light as possible)

- Think of three different words, any words which just come to your mind at the moment and make a simple story using these 3 words. Repeat untill you fall asleep.

If above does not help

- Say STOP untill you fall asleep

If above does not help

- Go to the kitchen and have a very small snack.
- Back to the bed think of three different words, any words which just come to your mind at the moment and make a simple story using these 3 words. Repeat untill you fall asleep.
- If above does not help think of three different words, any words which just come to your mind at the moment and make a simple story using these 3 words. Repeat untill you fall asleep.

***

Day 4

Morning

* Say STOP when the voices you hear in your head become too loud to hear your own thoughts.

* If above does not help to stop the voices, just turn your attention away from the voices. The best way to turn your attention away from the voices in your head is by doing one of your favorite occupations. Do not be ashamed of any occupation to turn your attention away from the voices in your head. ALWAYS be busy with your favorite occupation when unsupportable voices come to your head.

* Be careful to keep for yourself these of your believes which are found to be strange by the people.

* CONTROL what you say. Say only things which are not strange for the people. You surely already know which of your believes are found to be strange by the people.

* If you do not know yet which of your believes are found to be strange by the people, OBSERVE how people react on what you say. If you see that people are ALERTED by your believes, it means your believes are strange. From now on AVOID presenting such believes.

* Think of three different words, any words which just come to your mind at the moment and make a simple story using these 3 words. Repeat 3 times.

* Try to concentrate on an object close to you, any object. What do you feel when looking at the object? What thoughts come to your mind when looking at the object?

* Small physical excercise (10 min)

* Small breakfast.

* Nice talk (no complaints, no problematic questions) 10 min. When nobody to talk with, phone or internet conversation oral or written.

* Walk 15 min.

* If you hear voices which are not heard by other people, ask yourself if it is possible to ignore the voices.

Yes

Great! In such a case continue ignoring them.

No

You have to learn to ignore the voices.

This Guide will teach you to ignore the voices.

Remember: even if you cannot stop the voices, the voices cannot stop you to live a normal life.

If you believe in things which other people consider strange, try to keep your strange believes for yourself. Everybody has to make the selection of what can be told to other people and what must be private. Believe me, many people have strange believes. Even much stranger than yours. And they are not considered to be sick. Why? Because they keep their strange believes for themselves. That is the secret.

***

Afternoon

* Think of three different words, any words which just come to your mind at the moment and make a simple story using these 3 words. Repeat 3 times.

* Try to concentrate on an object close to you, any object. What do you feel when looking at the object? What thoughts come to your mind when looking at the object?

* Dinner and half an hour break (you can sleep).

* Nice talk (no complaints) 15 min. When nobody to talk with, phone or internet conversation oral or written.

* Walk 20 min.

* If you hear voices which are not heard by other people, ask yourself if it is possible to ignore them.

Yes

Great! In such a case continue ignoring them.

No

You have to learn to ignore the voices.

This Guide will teach you to ignore the voices.

Remember: even if you cannot stop the voices, the voices cannot stop you to live a normal life.

If you believe in things which other people consider strange, try to keep your strange believes for yourself. Everybody has to make the selection of what can be told to other people and what must be private. Believe me, many people have strange believes. Even much stranger than yours. And they are not considered to be sick. Why? Because they keep their strange believes for themselves. That is the secret.

***

Evening

- Think of three different words, any words which just come to your mind at the moment and make a simple story using these 3 words. Repeat 3 times.
    - Try to concentrate on an object close to you, any object. What do you feel when looking at the object? What thoughts come to your mind when looking at the object?
    - Small supper.

- Nice talk (no complaints) 10 min. When nobody to talk with, phone or internet conversation oral or written.
- Walk 10 min.
- If you hear voices which are not heard by other people, ask yourself if it is possible to ignore them.

Yes

Great! In such a case continue ignoring them.

No

You have to learn to ignore the voices.

This Guide will teach you to ignore the voices.

Remember: even if you cannot stop the voices, the voices cannot stop you to live a normal life.

If you believe in things which other people consider strange, try to keep your strange believes for yourself. Everybody has to make the selection of what can be told to other people and what must be private. Believe me, many people have strange believes. Even much stranger than yours. And they are not considered to be sick. Why? Because they keep their strange believes for themselves. That is the secret.

***

Night

Before sleep

- Take a shower (warm water) 1 min.
- Small physical excercise 3 min.

In Bed

- Repeat STOP (10 times if you hear the voices.
- Think of three different words, any words which just come to your mind at the moment and make a simple story using these 3 words. Repeat untill you fall asleep.

If you cannot fall asleep

- Think of three different words, any words which just come to your mind at the moment and make a simple story using these 3 words. Repeat untill you fall asleep.

If above does not help

- Stand up and go to the toilet (when possible with as little light as possible)
- Think of three different words, any words which just come to your mind at the moment and make a simple story using these 3 words. Repeat untill you fall asleep.

If above does not help

- Say STOP untill you fall asleep

If above does not help

- Go to the kitchen and have a very small snack.
- Back to the bed think of three different words, any words which just come to your mind at the moment and make a simple story using these 3 words. Repeat untill you fall asleep.
- If above does not help think of three different words, any words which just come to your mind at the moment and make a simple story using these 3 words. Repeat untill you fall asleep.

***

Day 5

Morning

* Say STOP when the voices you hear in your head become too loud to hear your own thoughts.

* If above does not help to stop the voices, just turn your attention away from the voices. The best way to turn your attention away from the voices in your head is by doing one of your favorite occupations. Do not be ashamed of any occupation to turn your attention away

from the voices in your head. ALWAYS be busy with your favorite occupation when unsupportable voices come to your head.

* Be careful to keep for yourself these of your believes which are found to be strange by the people.

* CONTROL what you say. Say only things which are not strange for the people. You surely already know which of your believes are found to be strange by the people.

* If you do not know yet which of your believes are found to be strange by the people, OBSERVE how people react on what you say. If you see that people are ALERTED by your believes, it means your believes are strange. From now on AVOID presenting such believes.

* Think of three different words, any words which just come to your mind at the moment and make a simple story using these 3 words. Repeat 3 times.

* Try to concentrate on an object close to you, any object. What do you feel when looking at the object? What thoughts come to your mind when looking at the object?

* Small physical excercise (10 min)

* Small breakfast.

* Nice talk (no complaints, no problematic questions) 10 min. When nobody to talk with, phone or internet conversation oral or written.

* Walk 15 min.

* If you hear voices which are not heard by other people, ask yourself if it is possible to ignore the voices.

Yes

Great! In such a case continue ignoring them.

No

You have to learn to ignore the voices.

This Guide will teach you to ignore the voices.

Remember: even if you cannot stop the voices, the voices cannot stop you to live a normal life.

If you believe in things which other people consider strange, try to keep your strange believes for yourself. Everybody has to make the selection of what can be told to other people and what must be private. Believe me, many people have strange believes. Even much stranger than yours. And they are not considered to be sick. Why? Because they keep their strange believes for themselves. That is the secret.

***

Afternoon

* Think of three different words, any words which just come to your mind at the moment and make a simple story using these 3 words. Repeat 3 times.

* Try to concentrate on an object close to you, any object. What do you feel when looking at the object? What thoughts come to your mind when looking at the object?

* Dinner and half an hour break (you can sleep).

* Nice talk (no complaints) 15 min. When nobody to talk with, phone or internet conversation oral or written.

* Walk 20 min.

* If you hear voices which are not heard by other people, ask yourself if it is possible to ignore them.

Yes

Great! In such a case continue ignoring them.

No

You have to learn to ignore the voices.

This Guide will teach you to ignore the voices.

Remember: even if you cannot stop the voices, the voices cannot stop you to live a normal life.

If you believe in things which other people consider strange, try to keep your strange believes for yourself. Everybody has to make the selection of what can be told to other people and what must be private. Believe me, many people have strange believes. Even much stranger than yours. And they are not considered to be sick. Why? Because they keep their strange believes for themselves. That is the secret.

***

Evening

- Think of three different words, any words which just come to your mind at the moment and make a simple story using these 3 words. Repeat 3 times.
  - Try to concentrate on an object close to you, any object. What do you feel when looking at the object? What thoughts come to your mind when looking at the object?
  - Small supper.

- Nice talk (no complaints) 10 min. When nobody to talk with, phone or internet conversation oral or written.
- Walk 10 min.
- If you hear voices which are not heard by other people, ask yourself if it is possible to ignore them.

Yes

Great! In such a case continue ignoring them.

No

You have to learn to ignore the voices.

This Guide will teach you to ignore the voices.

Remember: even if you cannot stop the voices, the voices cannot stop you to live a normal life.

If you believe in things which other people consider strange, try to keep your strange believes for yourself. Everybody has to make the selection of what can be told to other people and what must be private. Believe me, many people have strange believes. Even much stranger than yours. And they are not considered to be sick. Why? Because they keep their strange believes for themselves. That is the secret.

***

Night

Before sleep

- Take a shower (warm water) 1 min.
- Small physical excercise 3 min.

In Bed

- Repeat STOP (10 times if you hear the voices.
- Think of three different words, any words which just come to your mind at the moment and make a simple story using these 3 words. Repeat untill you fall asleep.

If you cannot fall asleep

- Think of three different words, any words which just come to your mind at the moment and make a simple story using these 3 words. Repeat untill you fall asleep.

If above does not help

- Stand up and go to the toilet (when possible with as little light as possible)
- Think of three different words, any words which just come to your mind at the moment and make a simple story using these 3 words. Repeat untill you fall asleep.

If above does not help

- Say STOP untill you fall asleep

If above does not help

- Go to the kitchen and have a very small snack.
- Back to the bed think of three different words, any words which just come to your mind at the moment and make a simple story using these 3 words. Repeat untill you fall asleep.
- If above does not help think of three different words, any words which just come to your mind at the moment and make a simple story using these 3 words. Repeat untill you fall asleep.

***

Day 6

Morning

* Say STOP when the voices you hear in your head become too loud to hear your own thoughts.

* If above does not help to stop the voices, just turn your attention away from the voices. The best way to turn your attention away from the voices in your head is by doing one of your favorite occupations. Do not be ashamed of any occupation to turn your attention away

from the voices in your head. ALWAYS be busy with your favorite occupation when unsupportable voices come to your head.

* Be careful to keep for yourself these of your believes which are found to be strange by the people.

* CONTROL what you say. Say only things which are not strange for the people. You surely already know which of your believes are found to be strange by the people.

* If you do not know yet which of your believes are found to be strange by the people, OBSERVE how people react on what you say. If you see that people are ALERTED by your believes, it means your believes are strange. From now on AVOID presenting such believes.

* Think of three different words, any words which just come to your mind at the moment and make a simple story using these 3 words. Repeat 3 times.

* Try to concentrate on an object close to you, any object. What do you feel when looking at the object? What thoughts come to your mind when looking at the object?

* Small physical excercise (10 min)

* Small breakfast.

* Nice talk (no complaints, no problematic questions) 10 min. When nobody to talk with, phone or internet conversation oral or written.

* Walk 15 min.

* If you hear voices which are not heard by other people, ask yourself if it is possible to ignore the voices.

Yes

Great! In such a case continue ignoring them.

No

You have to learn to ignore the voices.

This Guide will teach you to ignore the voices.

Remember: even if you cannot stop the voices, the voices cannot stop you to live a normal life.

If you believe in things which other people consider strange, try to keep your strange believes for yourself. Everybody has to make the selection of what can be told to other people and what must be private. Believe me, many people have strange believes. Even much stranger than yours. And they are not considered to be sick. Why? Because they keep their strange believes for themselves. That is the secret.

***

Afternoon

* Think of three different words, any words which just come to your mind at the moment and make a simple story using these 3 words. Repeat 3 times.

* Try to concentrate on an object close to you, any object. What do you feel when looking at the object? What thoughts come to your mind when looking at the object?

* Dinner and half an hour break (you can sleep).

* Nice talk (no complaints) 15 min. When nobody to talk with, phone or internet conversation oral or written.

* Walk 20 min.

* If you hear voices which are not heard by other people, ask yourself if it is possible to ignore them.

Yes

Great! In such a case continue ignoring them.

No

You have to learn to ignore the voices.

This Guide will teach you to ignore the voices.

Remember: even if you cannot stop the voices, the voices cannot stop you to live a normal life.

If you believe in things which other people consider strange, try to keep your strange believes for yourself. Everybody has to make the selection of what can be told to other people and what must be private. Believe me, many people have strange believes. Even much stranger than yours. And they are not considered to be sick. Why? Because they keep their strange believes for themselves. That is the secret.

***

Evening

- Think of three different words, any words which just come to your mind at the moment and make a simple story using these 3 words. Repeat 3 times.
  - Try to concentrate on an object close to you, any object. What do you feel when looking at the object? What thoughts come to your mind when looking at the object?
  - Small supper.

- Nice talk (no complaints) 10 min. When nobody to talk with, phone or internet conversation oral or written.
- Walk 10 min.
- If you hear voices which are not heard by other people, ask yourself if it is possible to ignore them.

Yes

Great! In such a case continue ignoring them.

No

You have to learn to ignore the voices.

This Guide will teach you to ignore the voices.

Remember: even if you cannot stop the voices, the voices cannot stop you to live a normal life.

If you believe in things which other people consider strange, try to keep your strange believes for yourself. Everybody has to make the selection of what can be told to other people and what must be private. Believe me, many people have strange believes. Even much stranger than yours. And they are not considered to be sick. Why? Because they keep their strange believes for themselves. That is the secret.

***

Night

Before sleep

- Take a shower (warm water) 1 min.
- Small physical excercise 3 min.

In Bed

- Repeat STOP (10 times if you hear the voices.
- Think of three different words, any words which just come to your mind at the moment and make a simple story using these 3 words. Repeat untill you fall asleep.

If you cannot fall asleep

- Think of three different words, any words which just come to your mind at the moment and make a simple story using these 3 words. Repeat untill you fall asleep.

If above does not help

- Stand up and go to the toilet (when possible with as little light as possible)
- Think of three different words, any words which just come to your mind at the moment and make a simple story using these 3 words. Repeat untill you fall asleep.

If above does not help

- Say STOP untill you fall asleep

If above does not help

- Go to the kitchen and have a very small snack.
- Back to the bed think of three different words, any words which just come to your mind at the moment and make a simple story using these 3 words. Repeat untill you fall asleep.
- If above does not help think of three different words, any words which just come to your mind at the moment and make a simple story using these 3 words. Repeat untill you fall asleep.

***

Day 7

Morning

* Say STOP when the voices you hear in your head become too loud to hear your own thoughts.

* If above does not help to stop the voices, just turn your attention away from the voices. The best way to turn your attention away from the voices in your head is by doing one of your favorite occupations. Do not be ashamed of any occupation to turn your attention away

from the voices in your head. ALWAYS be busy with your favorite occupation when unsupportable voices come to your head.

* Be careful to keep for yourself these of your believes which are found to be strange by the people.

* CONTROL what you say. Say only things which are not strange for the people. You surely already know which of your believes are found to be strange by the people.

* If you do not know yet which of your believes are found to be strange by the people, OBSERVE how people react on what you say. If you see that people are ALERTED by your believes, it means your believes are strange. From now on AVOID presenting such believes.

* Think of three different words, any words which just come to your mind at the moment and make a simple story using these 3 words. Repeat 3 times.

* Try to concentrate on an object close to you, any object. What do you feel when looking at the object? What thoughts come to your mind when looking at the object?

* Small physical excercise (10 min)

* Small breakfast.

* Nice talk (no complaints, no problematic questions) 10 min. When nobody to talk with, phone or internet conversation oral or written.

* Walk 15 min.

* If you hear voices which are not heard by other people, ask yourself if it is possible to ignore the voices.

Yes

Great! In such a case continue ignoring them.

No

You have to learn to ignore the voices.

This Guide will teach you to ignore the voices.

Remember: even if you cannot stop the voices, the voices cannot stop you to live a normal life.

If you believe in things which other people consider strange, try to keep your strange believes for yourself. Everybody has to make the selection of what can be told to other people and what must be private. Believe me, many people have strange believes. Even much stranger than yours. And they are not considered to be sick. Why? Because they keep their strange believes for themselves. That is the secret.

***

Afternoon

* Think of three different words, any words which just come to your mind at the moment and make a simple story using these 3 words. Repeat 3 times.

* Try to concentrate on an object close to you, any object. What do you feel when looking at the object? What thoughts come to your mind when looking at the object?

* Dinner and half an hour break (you can sleep).

* Nice talk (no complaints) 15 min. When nobody to talk with, phone or internet conversation oral or written.

* Walk 20 min.

* If you hear voices which are not heard by other people, ask yourself if it is possible to ignore them.

Yes

Great! In such a case continue ignoring them.

No

You have to learn to ignore the voices.

This Guide will teach you to ignore the voices.

Remember: even if you cannot stop the voices, the voices cannot stop you to live a normal life.

If you believe in things which other people consider strange, try to keep your strange believes for yourself. Everybody has to make the selection of what can be told to other people and what must be private. Believe me, many people have strange believes. Even much stranger than yours. And they are not considered to be sick. Why? Because they keep their strange believes for themselves. That is the secret.

***

Evening

- Think of three different words, any words which just come to your mind at the moment and make a simple story using these 3 words. Repeat 3 times.
  - Try to concentrate on an object close to you, any object. What do you feel when looking at the object? What thoughts come to your mind when looking at the object?
  - Small supper.

- Nice talk (no complaints) 10 min. When nobody to talk with, phone or internet conversation oral or written.
- Walk 10 min.
- If you hear voices which are not heard by other people, ask yourself if it is possible to ignore them.

Yes

Great! In such a case continue ignoring them.

No

You have to learn to ignore the voices.

This Guide will teach you to ignore the voices.

Remember: even if you cannot stop the voices, the voices cannot stop you to live a normal life.

If you believe in things which other people consider strange, try to keep your strange believes for yourself. Everybody has to make the selection of what can be told to other people and what must be private. Believe me, many people have strange believes. Even much stranger than yours. And they are not considered to be sick. Why? Because they keep their strange believes for themselves. That is the secret.

***

Night

Before sleep

- Take a shower (warm water) 1 min.
- Small physical excercise 3 min.

In Bed

- Repeat STOP (10 times if you hear the voices.
- Think of three different words, any words which just come to your mind at the moment and make a simple story using these 3 words. Repeat untill you fall asleep.

If you cannot fall asleep

- Think of three different words, any words which just come to your mind at the moment and make a simple story using these 3 words. Repeat untill you fall asleep.

If above does not help

- Stand up and go to the toilet (when possible with as little light as possible)
- Think of three different words, any words which just come to your mind at the moment and make a simple story using these 3 words. Repeat untill you fall asleep.

If above does not help

- Say STOP untill you fall asleep

If above does not help

- Go to the kitchen and have a very small snack.
- Back to the bed think of three different words, any words which just come to your mind at the moment and make a simple story using these 3 words. Repeat untill you fall asleep.
- If above does not help think of three different words, any words which just come to your mind at the moment and make a simple story using these 3 words. Repeat untill you fall asleep.

***

Week Two

***

Day 1

Morning

* Say STOP when the voices you hear in your head become too loud to hear your own thoughts.

* If above does not help to stop the voices, just turn your attention away from the voices. The best way to turn your attention away from the voices in your head is by doing one of your favorite occupations. Do not be ashamed of any occupation to turn your attention away from the voices in your head. ALWAYS be busy with your favorite occupation when unsupportable voices come to your head.

* Be careful to keep for yourself these of your believes which are found to be strange by the people.

* CONTROL what you say. Say only things which are not strange for the people. You surely already know which of your believes are found to be strange by the people.

* If you do not know yet which of your believes are found to be strange by the people, OBSERVE how people react on what you say. If you see that people are ALERTED by your believes, it means your believes are strange. From now on AVOID presenting such believes.

* Think of three different words, any words which just come to your mind at the moment and make a simple story using these 3 words. Repeat 3 times.

* Try to concentrate on an object close to you, any object. What do you feel when looking at the object? What thoughts come to your mind when looking at the object?

* Small physical excercise (10 min)

* Small breakfast.

* Nice talk (no complaints, no problematic questions) 10 min. When nobody to talk with, phone or internet conversation oral or written.

* Walk 15 min.

* If you hear voices which are not heard by other people, ask yourself if it is possible to ignore the voices.

Yes

Great! In such a case continue ignoring them.

No

You have to learn to ignore the voices.

This Guide will teach you to ignore the voices.

Remember: even if you cannot stop the voices, the voices cannot stop you to live a normal life.

If you believe in things which other people consider strange, try to keep your strange believes for yourself. Everybody has to make the selection of what can be told to other people and what must be private. Believe me, many people have strange believes. Even much stranger than yours. And they are not considered to be sick. Why? Because they keep their strange believes for themselves. That is the secret.

***

Afternoon

* Think of three different words, any words which just come to your mind at the moment and make a simple story using these 3 words. Repeat 3 times.

* Try to concentrate on an object close to you, any object. What do you feel when looking at the object? What thoughts come to your mind when looking at the object?

* Dinner and half an hour break (you can sleep).

* Nice talk (no complaints) 15 min. When nobody to talk with, phone or internet conversation oral or written.

* Walk 20 min.

* If you hear voices which are not heard by other people, ask yourself if it is possible to ignore them.

Yes

Great! In such a case continue ignoring them.

No

You have to learn to ignore the voices.

This Guide will teach you to ignore the voices.

Remember: even if you cannot stop the voices, the voices cannot stop you to live a normal life.

If you believe in things which other people consider strange, try to keep your strange believes for yourself. Everybody has to make the selection of what can be told to other people and what must be private. Believe me, many people have strange believes. Even much stranger than yours. And they are not considered to be sick. Why? Because they keep their strange believes for themselves. That is the secret.

***

Evening

- Think of three different words, any words which just come to your mind at the moment and make a simple story using these 3 words. Repeat 3 times.
  - Try to concentrate on an object close to you, any object. What do you feel when looking at the object? What thoughts come to your mind when looking at the object?
  - Small supper.

- Nice talk (no complaints) 10 min. When nobody to talk with, phone or internet conversation oral or written.
- Walk 10 min.
- If you hear voices which are not heard by other people, ask yourself if it is possible to ignore them.

Yes

Great! In such a case continue ignoring them.

No

You have to learn to ignore the voices.

This Guide will teach you to ignore the voices.

Remember: even if you cannot stop the voices, the voices cannot stop you to live a normal life.

If you believe in things which other people consider strange, try to keep your strange believes for yourself. Everybody has to make the selection of what can be told to other people and what must be private. Believe me, many people have strange believes. Even much stranger than yours. And they are not considered to be sick. Why? Because they keep their strange believes for themselves. That is the secret.

***

Night

Before sleep

- Take a shower (warm water) 1 min.
- Small physical excercise 3 min.

In Bed

- Repeat STOP (10 times if you hear the voices.
- Think of three different words, any words which just come to your mind at the moment and make a simple story using these 3 words. Repeat untill you fall asleep.

If you cannot fall asleep

- Think of three different words, any words which just come to your mind at the moment and make a simple story using these 3 words. Repeat untill you fall asleep.

If above does not help

- Stand up and go to the toilet (when possible with as little light as possible)
- Think of three different words, any words which just come to your mind at the moment and make a simple story using these 3 words. Repeat untill you fall asleep.

If above does not help

- Say STOP untill you fall asleep

If above does not help

- Go to the kitchen and have a very small snack.
- Back to the bed think of three different words, any words which just come to your mind at the moment and make a simple story using these 3 words. Repeat untill you fall asleep.
- If above does not help think of three different words, any words which just come to your mind at the moment and make a simple story using these 3 words. Repeat untill you fall asleep.

***

Day 2

Morning

- Say STOP when the voices you hear in your head become too loud to hear your own thoughts.
- If above does not help to stop the voices, just turn your attention away from the voices. The best way to turn your attention away from the voices in your head is by doing one of your favorite occupations. Do not be ashamed of any occupation to turn your attention away from the

voices in your head. ALWAYS be busy with your favorite occupation when unsupportable voices come to your head.
- Be careful to keep for yourself these of your believes which are found to be strange by the people.
- CONTROL what you say. Say only things which are not strange for the people. You surely already know which of your believes are found to be strange by the people.
- If you do not know yet which of your believes are found to be strange by the people, OBSERVE how people react on what you say. If you see that people are ALERTED by your believes, it means your believes are strange. From now on AVOID presenting such believes.
- Think of three different words, any words which just come to your mind at the moment and make a simple story using these 3 words. Repeat 3 times.
- Try to concentrate on an object close to you, any object. What do you feel when looking at the object? What thoughts come to your mind when looking at the object?
- Small physical excercise (10 min)
- Small breakfast.

- Nice talk (no complaints, no problematic questions) 10 min. When nobody to talk with, phone or internet conversation oral or written.
- Walk 15 min.
- If you hear voices which are not heard by other people, ask yourself if it is possible to ignore the voices.

Yes

Great! In such a case continue ignoring them.
No
You have to learn to ignore the voices.
This Guide will teach you to ignore the voices.
Remember: even if you cannot stop the voices, the voices cannot stop you to live a normal life.

If you believe in things which other people consider strange, try to keep your strange believes for yourself. Everybody has to make the selection of what can be told to other people and what must be private. Believe me, many people have strange believes. Even much stranger than yours. And they are not considered to be sick. Why? Because they keep their strange believes for themselves. That is the secret.

***

Afternoon
- Think of three different words, any words which just come to your mind at the moment and make a simple story using these 3 words. Repeat 3 times.
- Try to concentrate on an object close to you, any object. What do you feel when looking at the object? What thoughts come to your mind when looking at the object?
- Dinner and half an hour break (you can sleep).
- Nice talk (no complaints) 15 min. When nobody to talk with, phone or internet conversation oral or written.
- Walk 20 min.
- If you hear voices which are not heard by other people, ask yourself if it is possible to ignore them.

  Yes

  Great! In such a case continue ignoring them.

  No

  You have to learn to ignore the voices.

  This Guide will teach you to ignore the voices. Remember: even if you cannot stop the voices, the voices cannot stop you to live a normal life.

- If you believe in things which other people consider strange, try to keep your strange believes for yourself. Everybody has to make the selection of what can be told to other people and what must be private. Believe me, many people have strange believes. Even much stranger than yours. And they are not considered to be sick. Why? Because they keep their strange believes for themselves. That is the secret.

***

Evening

- Think of three different words, any words which just come to your mind at the moment and make a simple story using these 3 words. Repeat 3 times.
- Try to concentrate on an object close to you, any object. What do you feel when looking at the object? What thoughts come to your mind when looking at the object?
- Small supper.

- Nice talk (no complaints) 10 min. When nobody to talk with, phone or internet conversation oral or written.
- Walk 10 min.
- If you hear voices which are not heard by other people, ask yourself if it is possible to ignore them.

  Yes

  Great! In such a case continue ignoring them.

No

You have to learn to ignore the voices.

This Guide will teach you to ignore the voices.

> Remember: even if you cannot stop the voices, the voices cannot stop you to live a normal life.
>
> If you believe in things which other people consider strange, try to keep your strange believes for yourself. Everybody has to make the selection of what can be told to other people and what must be private. Believe me, many people have strange believes. Even much stranger than yours. And they are not considered to be sick. Why? Because they keep their strange believes for themselves. That is the secret.

***

Night

Before sleep

- Take a shower (warm water) 1 min.
- Small physical excercise 3 min.

In Bed

- Repeat STOP (10 times if you hear the voices.
- Think of three different words, any words which just come to your mind at the moment and make a simple story using these 3 words. Repeat untill you fall asleep.
- If you cannot fall asleep
- Think of three different words, any words which just come to your mind at the moment and make a simple story using these 3 words. Repeat untill you fall asleep.
- If above does not help
- Stand up and go to the toilet (when possible with as little light as possible)
- Think of three different words, any words which just come to your mind at the moment and make a simple story using these 3 words. Repeat untill you fall asleep.
- If above does not help
- Say STOP untill you fall asleep

- If above does not help
- Go to the kitchen and have a very small snack.
- Back to the bed think of three different words, any words which just come to your mind at the moment and make a simple story using these 3 words. Repeat untill you fall asleep.
- If above does not help think of three different words, any words which just come to your mind at the moment and make a simple story using these 3 words. Repeat untill you fall asleep.

***

Day 3

Morning

* Say STOP when the voices you hear in your head become too loud to hear your own thoughts.

* If above does not help to stop the voices, just turn your attention away from the voices. The best way to turn your attention away from the voices in your head is by doing one of your favorite occupations. Do not be ashamed of any occupation to turn your attention away from the voices in your head. ALWAYS be busy with your favorite occupation when unsupportable voices come to your head.

* Be careful to keep for yourself these of your believes which are found to be strange by the people.
* CONTROL what you say. Say only things which are not strange for the people. You surely already know which of your believes are found to be strange by the people.
* If you do not know yet which of your believes are found to be strange by the people, OBSERVE how people react on what you say. If you see that people are ALERTED by your believes, it means your believes are strange. From now on AVOID presenting such believes.
* Think of three different words, any words which just come to your mind at the moment and make a simple story using these 3 words. Repeat 3 times.
* Try to concentrate on an object close to you, any object. What do you feel when looking at the object? What thoughts come to your mind when looking at the object?
* Small physical excercise (10 min)
* Small breakfast.
* Nice talk (no complaints, no problematic questions) 10 min. When nobody to talk with, phone or internet conversation oral or written.

* Walk 15 min.
* If you hear voices which are not heard by other people, ask yourself if it is possible to ignore the voices.

Yes

Great! In such a case continue ignoring them.

No

You have to learn to ignore the voices.
This Guide will teach you to ignore the voices. Remember: even if you cannot stop the voices, the voices cannot stop you to live a normal life.

If you believe in things which other people consider strange, try to keep your strange believes for yourself. Everybody has to make the selection of what can be told to other people and what must be private. Believe me, many people have strange believes. Even much stranger than yours. And they are not considered to be sick. Why? Because they keep their strange believes for themselves. That is the secret.

***

Afternoon

* Think of three different words, any words which just come to your mind at the moment and make a simple story using these 3 words. Repeat 3 times.
* Try to concentrate on an object close to you, any object. What do you feel when looking at the object? What thoughts come to your mind when looking at the object?
* Dinner and half an hour break (you can sleep).
* Nice talk (no complaints) 15 min. When nobody to talk with, phone or internet conversation oral or written.
* Walk 20 min.
* If you hear voices which are not heard by other people, ask yourself if it is possible to ignore them.

Yes

Great! In such a case continue ignoring them.

No

You have to learn to ignore the voices.
This Guide will teach you to ignore the voices.
Remember: even if you cannot stop the voices, the voices cannot stop you to live a normal life.

If you believe in things which other people consider strange, try to keep your strange

believes for yourself. Everybody has to make the selection of what can be told to other people and what must be private. Believe me, many people have strange believes. Even much stranger than yours. And they are not considered to be sick. Why? Because they keep their strange believes for themselves. That is the secret.

***

Evening

- Think of three different words, any words which just come to your mind at the moment and make a simple story using these 3 words. Repeat 3 times.
- Try to concentrate on an object close to you, any object. What do you feel when looking at the object? What thoughts come to your mind when looking at the object?
- Small supper.
- Nice talk (no complaints) 10 min. When nobody to talk with, phone or internet conversation oral or written.
- Walk 10 min.

- If you hear voices which are not heard by other people, ask yourself if it is possible to ignore them.

Yes

Great! In such a case continue ignoring them.

No

You have to learn to ignore the voices. This Guide will teach you to ignore the voices. Remember: even if you cannot stop the voices, the voices cannot stop you to live a normal life.

If you believe in things which other people consider strange, try to keep your strange believes for yourself. Everybody has to make the selection of what can be told to other people and what must be private. Believe me, many people have strange believes. Even much stranger than yours. And they are not considered to be sick. Why? Because they keep their strange believes for themselves. That is the secret.

***

Night

Before sleep

- Take a shower (warm water) 1 min.
- Small physical excercise 3 min.

In Bed
- Repeat STOP (10 times if you hear the voices.
- Think of three different words, any words which just come to your mind at the moment and make a simple story using these 3 words. Repeat untill you fall asleep.

If you cannot fall asleep
- Think of three different words, any words which just come to your mind at the moment and make a simple story using these 3 words. Repeat untill you fall asleep.

If above does not help
- Stand up and go to the toilet (when possible with as little light as possible)
- Think of three different words, any words which just come to your mind at the moment and make a simple story using these 3 words. Repeat untill you fall asleep.

If above does not help
- Say STOP untill you fall asleep

If above does not help
- Go to the kitchen and have a very small snack.
- Back to the bed think of three different words, any words which just come to your mind at the moment and make a simple story using these 3 words. Repeat untill you fall asleep.

- If above does not help think of three different words, any words which just come to your mind at the moment and make a simple story using these 3 words. Repeat untill you fall asleep.

***

Day 4

Morning

* Say STOP when the voices you hear in your head become too loud to hear your own thoughts.
* If above does not help to stop the voices, just turn your attention away from the voices. The best way to turn your attention away from the voices in your head is by doing one of your favorite occupations. Do not be ashamed of any occupation to turn your attention away from the voices in your head. ALWAYS be busy with your favorite occupation when unsupportable voices come to your head.
* Be careful to keep for yourself these of your believes which are found to be strange by the people.
* CONTROL what you say. Say only things which are not strange for the people. You surely

already know which of your believes are found to be strange by the people.
* If you do not know yet which of your believes are found to be strange by the people, OBSERVE how people react on what you say. If you see that people are ALERTED by your believes, it means your believes are strange. From now on AVOID presenting such believes.
* Think of three different words, any words which just come to your mind at the moment and make a simple story using these 3 words. Repeat 3 times.
* Try to concentrate on an object close to you, any object. What do you feel when looking at the object? What thoughts come to your mind when looking at the object?
* Small physical excercise (10 min)
* Small breakfast.
* Nice talk (no complaints, no problematic questions) 10 min. When nobody to talk with, phone or internet conversation oral or written.
* Walk 15 min.
* If you hear voices which are not heard by other people, ask yourself if it is possible to ignore the voices.
Yes

Great! In such a case continue ignoring them.
No
You have to learn to ignore the voices.
This Guide will teach you to ignore the voices.
Remember: even if you cannot stop the voices, the voices cannot stop you to live a normal life.

If you believe in things which other people consider strange, try to keep your strange believes for yourself. Everybody has to make the selection of what can be told to other people and what must be private. Believe me, many people have strange believes. Even much stranger than yours. And they are not considered to be sick. Why? Because they keep their strange believes for themselves. That is the secret.

***

Afternoon
* Think of three different words, any words which just come to your mind at the moment and make a simple story using these 3 words. Repeat 3 times.
* Try to concentrate on an object close to you, any object. What do you feel when looking at

the object? What thoughts come to your mind when looking at the object?
* Dinner and half an hour break (you can sleep).
* Nice talk (no complaints) 15 min. When nobody to talk with, phone or internet conversation oral or written.
* Walk 20 min.
* If you hear voices which are not heard by other people, ask yourself if it is possible to ignore them.
Yes
Great! In such a case continue ignoring them.
No
You have to learn to ignore the voices.
This Guide will teach you to ignore the voices. Remember: even if you cannot stop the voices, the voices cannot stop you to live a normal life.

If you believe in things which other people consider strange, try to keep your strange believes for yourself. Everybody has to make the selection of what can be told to other people and what must be private. Believe me, many people have strange believes. Even much stranger than yours. And they are not considered to be sick. Why? Because they keep

their strange believes for themselves. That is the secret.

***

Evening

- Think of three different words, any words which just come to your mind at the moment and make a simple story using these 3 words. Repeat 3 times.
- Try to concentrate on an object close to you, any object. What do you feel when looking at the object? What thoughts come to your mind when looking at the object?
- Small supper.
- Nice talk (no complaints) 10 min. When nobody to talk with, phone or internet conversation oral or written.
- Walk 10 min.
- If you hear voices which are not heard by other people, ask yourself if it is possible to ignore them.

Yes

Great! In such a case continue ignoring them.

No

You have to learn to ignore the voices.
This Guide will teach you to ignore the voices.

Remember: even if you cannot stop the voices, the voices cannot stop you to live a normal life.

If you believe in things which other people consider strange, try to keep your strange believes for yourself. Everybody has to make the selection of what can be told to other people and what must be private. Believe me, many people have strange believes. Even much stranger than yours. And they are not considered to be sick. Why? Because they keep their strange believes for themselves. That is the secret.

***

Night

Before sleep
- Take a shower (warm water) 1 min.
- Small physical excercise 3 min.

In Bed
- Repeat STOP (10 times if you hear the voices.
- Think of three different words, any words which just come to your mind at the moment and make a simple story using these 3 words. Repeat untill you fall asleep.

If you cannot fall asleep

- Think of three different words, any words which just come to your mind at the moment and make a simple story using these 3 words. Repeat untill you fall asleep.

If above does not help
- Stand up and go to the toilet (when possible with as little light as possible)
- Think of three different words, any words which just come to your mind at the moment and make a simple story using these 3 words. Repeat untill you fall asleep.

If above does not help
- Say STOP untill you fall asleep

If above does not help
- Go to the kitchen and have a very small snack.
- Back to the bed think of three different words, any words which just come to your mind at the moment and make a simple story using these 3 words. Repeat untill you fall asleep.
- If above does not help think of three different words, any words which just come to your mind at the moment and make a simple story using these 3 words. Repeat untill you fall asleep.

***

Day 5

Morning
* Say STOP when the voices you hear in your head become too loud to hear your own thoughts.
* If above does not help to stop the voices, just turn your attention away from the voices. The best way to turn your attention away from the voices in your head is by doing one of your favorite occupations. Do not be ashamed of any occupation to turn your attention away from the voices in your head. ALWAYS be busy with your favorite occupation when unsupportable voices come to your head.
* Be careful to keep for yourself these of your believes which are found to be strange by the people.
* CONTROL what you say. Say only things which are not strange for the people. You surely already know which of your believes are found to be strange by the people.
* If you do not know yet which of your believes are found to be strange by the people, OBSERVE how people react on what you say. If you see that people are ALERTED by your believes, it means your believes are strange. From now on AVOID presenting such believes.

* Think of three different words, any words which just come to your mind at the moment and make a simple story using these 3 words. Repeat 3 times.
* Try to concentrate on an object close to you, any object. What do you feel when looking at the object? What thoughts come to your mind when looking at the object?
* Small physical excercise (10 min)
* Small breakfast.
* Nice talk (no complaints, no problematic questions) 10 min. When nobody to talk with, phone or internet conversation oral or written.
* Walk 15 min.
* If you hear voices which are not heard by other people, ask yourself if it is possible to ignore the voices.

Yes

Great! In such a case continue ignoring them.

No

You have to learn to ignore the voices.

This Guide will teach you to ignore the voices.

Remember: even if you cannot stop the voices, the voices cannot stop you to live a normal life.

If you believe in things which other people consider strange, try to keep your strange believes for yourself. Everybody has to make the selection of what can be told to other people and what must be private. Believe me, many people have strange believes. Even much stranger than yours. And they are not considered to be sick. Why? Because they keep their strange believes for themselves. That is the secret.

***

Afternoon
* Think of three different words, any words which just come to your mind at the moment and make a simple story using these 3 words. Repeat 3 times.
* Try to concentrate on an object close to you, any object. What do you feel when looking at the object? What thoughts come to your mind when looking at the object?
* Dinner and half an hour break (you can sleep).
* Nice talk (no complaints) 15 min. When nobody to talk with, phone or internet conversation oral or written.
* Walk 20 min.

* If you hear voices which are not heard by other people, ask yourself if it is possible to ignore them.
Yes
Great! In such a case continue ignoring them.
No
You have to learn to ignore the voices.
This Guide will teach you to ignore the voices.
Remember: even if you cannot stop the voices, the voices cannot stop you to live a normal life.

If you believe in things which other people consider strange, try to keep your strange believes for yourself. Everybody has to make the selection of what can be told to other people and what must be private. Believe me, many people have strange believes. Even much stranger than yours. And they are not considered to be sick. Why? Because they keep their strange believes for themselves. That is the secret.
***
Evening

- Think of three different words, any words which just come to your mind at the moment

and make a simple story using these 3 words. Repeat 3 times.
- Try to concentrate on an object close to you, any object. What do you feel when looking at the object? What thoughts come to your mind when looking at the object?
- Small supper.
- Nice talk (no complaints) 10 min. When nobody to talk with, phone or internet conversation oral or written.
- Walk 10 min.
- If you hear voices which are not heard by other people, ask yourself if it is possible to ignore them.

Yes

Great! In such a case continue ignoring them.

No

You have to learn to ignore the voices.
This Guide will teach you to ignore the voices.
Remember: even if you cannot stop the voices, the voices cannot stop you to live a normal life.

If you believe in things which other people consider strange, try to keep your strange believes for yourself. Everybody has to make the selection of what can be told to other people

and what must be private. Believe me, many people have strange believes. Even much stranger than yours. And they are not considered to be sick. Why? Because they keep their strange believes for themselves. That is the secret.

***

Night

Before sleep
- Take a shower (warm water) 1 min.
- Small physical excercise 3 min.

In Bed
- Repeat STOP (10 times if you hear the voices.
- Think of three different words, any words which just come to your mind at the moment and make a simple story using these 3 words. Repeat untill you fall asleep.

If you cannot fall asleep
- Think of three different words, any words which just come to your mind at the moment and make a simple story using these 3 words. Repeat untill you fall asleep.

If above does not help
- Stand up and go to the toilet (when possible with as little light as possible)

- Think of three different words, any words which just come to your mind at the moment and make a simple story using these 3 words. Repeat untill you fall asleep.

If above does not help
- Say STOP untill you fall asleep

If above does not help
- Go to the kitchen and have a very small snack.
- Back to the bed think of three different words, any words which just come to your mind at the moment and make a simple story using these 3 words. Repeat untill you fall asleep.
- If above does not help think of three different words, any words which just come to your mind at the moment and make a simple story using these 3 words. Repeat untill you fall asleep.

***

Day 6

Morning

* Say STOP when the voices you hear in your head become too loud to hear your own thoughts.

* If above does not help to stop the voices, just turn your attention away from the voices. The best way to turn your attention away from the

voices in your head is by doing one of your favorite occupations. Do not be ashamed of any occupation to turn your attention away from the voices in your head. ALWAYS be busy with your favorite occupation when unsupportable voices come to your head.

* Be careful to keep for yourself these of your believes which are found to be strange by the people.

* CONTROL what you say. Say only things which are not strange for the people. You surely already know which of your believes are found to be strange by the people.

* If you do not know yet which of your believes are found to be strange by the people, OBSERVE how people react on what you say. If you see that people are ALERTED by your believes, it means your believes are strange. From now on AVOID presenting such believes.

* Think of three different words, any words which just come to your mind at the moment and make a simple story using these 3 words. Repeat 3 times.

* Try to concentrate on an object close to you, any object. What do you feel when looking at

the object? What thoughts come to your mind when looking at the object?
* Small physical excercise (10 min)
* Small breakfast.
* Nice talk (no complaints, no problematic questions) 10 min. When nobody to talk with, phone or internet conversation oral or written.
* Walk 15 min.
* If you hear voices which are not heard by other people, ask yourself if it is possible to ignore the voices.

Yes

Great! In such a case continue ignoring them.

No

You have to learn to ignore the voices.
This Guide will teach you to ignore the voices.
Remember: even if you cannot stop the voices, the voices cannot stop you to live a normal life.

If you believe in things which other people consider strange, try to keep your strange believes for yourself. Everybody has to make the selection of what can be told to other people and what must be private. Believe me, many people have strange believes. Even much stranger than yours. And they are not

considered to be sick. Why? Because they keep their strange believes for themselves. That is the secret.

***

Afternoon
* Think of three different words, any words which just come to your mind at the moment and make a simple story using these 3 words. Repeat 3 times.
* Try to concentrate on an object close to you, any object. What do you feel when looking at the object? What thoughts come to your mind when looking at the object?
* Dinner and half an hour break (you can sleep).
* Nice talk (no complaints) 15 min. When nobody to talk with, phone or internet conversation oral or written.
* Walk 20 min.
* If you hear voices which are not heard by other people, ask yourself if it is possible to ignore them.
Yes
Great! In such a case continue ignoring them.
No
You have to learn to ignore the voices.

This Guide will teach you to ignore the voices. Remember: even if you cannot stop the voices, the voices cannot stop you to live a normal life.

If you believe in things which other people consider strange, try to keep your strange believes for yourself. Everybody has to make the selection of what can be told to other people and what must be private. Believe me, many people have strange believes. Even much stranger than yours. And they are not considered to be sick. Why? Because they keep their strange believes for themselves. That is the secret.

***

Evening

- Think of three different words, any words which just come to your mind at the moment and make a simple story using these 3 words. Repeat 3 times.
- Try to concentrate on an object close to you, any object. What do you feel when looking at the object? What thoughts come to your mind when looking at the object?
- Small supper.

- Nice talk (no complaints) 10 min. When nobody to talk with, phone or internet conversation oral or written.
- Walk 10 min.
- If you hear voices which are not heard by other people, ask yourself if it is possible to ignore them.

Yes

Great! In such a case continue ignoring them.

No

You have to learn to ignore the voices.
This Guide will teach you to ignore the voices.
Remember: even if you cannot stop the voices, the voices cannot stop you to live a normal life.

If you believe in things which other people consider strange, try to keep your strange believes for yourself. Everybody has to make the selection of what can be told to other people and what must be private. Believe me, many people have strange believes. Even much stranger than yours. And they are not considered to be sick. Why? Because they keep their strange believes for themselves. That is the secret.

***

Night

Before sleep
- Take a shower (warm water) 1 min.
- Small physical excercise 3 min.

In Bed
- Repeat STOP (10 times if you hear the voices.
- Think of three different words, any words which just come to your mind at the moment and make a simple story using these 3 words. Repeat untill you fall asleep.

If you cannot fall asleep
- Think of three different words, any words which just come to your mind at the moment and make a simple story using these 3 words. Repeat untill you fall asleep.

If above does not help
- Stand up and go to the toilet (when possible with as little light as possible)
- Think of three different words, any words which just come to your mind at the moment and make a simple story using these 3 words. Repeat untill you fall asleep.

If above does not help
- Say STOP untill you fall asleep

If above does not help
- Go to the kitchen and have a very small snack.

- Back to the bed think of three different words, any words which just come to your mind at the moment and make a simple story using these 3 words. Repeat untill you fall asleep.
- If above does not help think of three different words, any words which just come to your mind at the moment and make a simple story using these 3 words. Repeat untill you fall asleep.

***

Day 7

Morning

* Say STOP when the voices you hear in your head become too loud to hear your own thoughts.

* If above does not help to stop the voices, just turn your attention away from the voices. The best way to turn your attention away from the voices in your head is by doing one of your favorite occupations. Do not be ashamed of any occupation to turn your attention away from the voices in your head. ALWAYS be busy with your favorite occupation when unsupportable voices come to your head.

* Be careful to keep for yourself these of your believes which are found to be strange by the people.
* CONTROL what you say. Say only things which are not strange for the people. You surely already know which of your believes are found to be strange by the people.
* If you do not know yet which of your believes are found to be strange by the people, OBSERVE how people react on what you say. If you see that people are ALERTED by your believes, it means your believes are strange. From now on AVOID presenting such believes.
* Think of three different words, any words which just come to your mind at the moment and make a simple story using these 3 words. Repeat 3 times.
* Try to concentrate on an object close to you, any object. What do you feel when looking at the object? What thoughts come to your mind when looking at the object?
* Small physical excercise (10 min)
* Small breakfast.
* Nice talk (no complaints, no problematic questions) 10 min. When nobody to talk with, phone or internet conversation oral or written.

* Walk 15 min.
* If you hear voices which are not heard by other people, ask yourself if it is possible to ignore the voices.

Yes

Great! In such a case continue ignoring them.

No

You have to learn to ignore the voices.
This Guide will teach you to ignore the voices. Remember: even if you cannot stop the voices, the voices cannot stop you to live a normal life.

If you believe in things which other people consider strange, try to keep your strange believes for yourself. Everybody has to make the selection of what can be told to other people and what must be private. Believe me, many people have strange believes. Even much stranger than yours. And they are not considered to be sick. Why? Because they keep their strange believes for themselves. That is the secret.

***

Afternoon

* Think of three different words, any words which just come to your mind at the moment and make a simple story using these 3 words. Repeat 3 times.
* Try to concentrate on an object close to you, any object. What do you feel when looking at the object? What thoughts come to your mind when looking at the object?
* Dinner and half an hour break (you can sleep).
* Nice talk (no complaints) 15 min. When nobody to talk with, phone or internet conversation oral or written.
* Walk 20 min.
* If you hear voices which are not heard by other people, ask yourself if it is possible to ignore them.

Yes

Great! In such a case continue ignoring them.

No

You have to learn to ignore the voices.
This Guide will teach you to ignore the voices.
Remember: even if you cannot stop the voices, the voices cannot stop you to live a normal life.

If you believe in things which other people consider strange, try to keep your strange

believes for yourself. Everybody has to make the selection of what can be told to other people and what must be private. Believe me, many people have strange believes. Even much stranger than yours. And they are not considered to be sick. Why? Because they keep their strange believes for themselves. That is the secret.

***

Evening

- Think of three different words, any words which just come to your mind at the moment and make a simple story using these 3 words. Repeat 3 times.
- Try to concentrate on an object close to you, any object. What do you feel when looking at the object? What thoughts come to your mind when looking at the object?
- Small supper.
- Nice talk (no complaints) 10 min. When nobody to talk with, phone or internet conversation oral or written.
- Walk 10 min.

- If you hear voices which are not heard by other people, ask yourself if it is possible to ignore them.

Yes

Great! In such a case continue ignoring them.

No

You have to learn to ignore the voices.
This Guide will teach you to ignore the voices. Remember: even if you cannot stop the voices, the voices cannot stop you to live a normal life.

If you believe in things which other people consider strange, try to keep your strange believes for yourself. Everybody has to make the selection of what can be told to other people and what must be private. Believe me, many people have strange believes. Even much stranger than yours. And they are not considered to be sick. Why? Because they keep their strange believes for themselves. That is the secret.

***

Night

Before sleep

- Take a shower (warm water) 1 min.
- Small physical excercise 3 min.

In Bed
- Repeat STOP (10 times if you hear the voices.
- Think of three different words, any words which just come to your mind at the moment and make a simple story using these 3 words. Repeat untill you fall asleep.

If you cannot fall asleep
- Think of three different words, any words which just come to your mind at the moment and make a simple story using these 3 words. Repeat untill you fall asleep.

If above does not help
- Stand up and go to the toilet (when possible with as little light as possible)
- Think of three different words, any words which just come to your mind at the moment and make a simple story using these 3 words. Repeat untill you fall asleep.

If above does not help
- Say STOP untill you fall asleep

If above does not help
- Go to the kitchen and have a very small snack.
- Back to the bed think of three different words, any words which just come to your mind at the moment and make a simple story using these 3 words. Repeat untill you fall asleep.

- If above does not help think of three different words, any words which just come to your mind at the moment and make a simple story using these 3 words. Repeat untill you fall asleep.

***

Week Three

***

Day 1

Morning

* Say STOP when the voices you hear in your head become too loud to hear your own thoughts.
* If above does not help to stop the voices, just turn your attention away from the voices. The best way to turn your attention away from the voices in your head is by doing one of your favorite occupations. Do not be ashamed of any occupation to turn your attention away from the voices in your head. ALWAYS be busy with your favorite occupation when unsupportable voices come to your head.
* Be careful to keep for yourself these of your believes which are found to be strange by the people.

* CONTROL what you say. Say only things which are not strange for the people. You surely already know which of your believes are found to be strange by the people.
* If you do not know yet which of your believes are found to be strange by the people, OBSERVE how people react on what you say. If you see that people are ALERTED by your believes, it means your believes are strange. From now on AVOID presenting such believes.
* Think of three different words, any words which just come to your mind at the moment and make a simple story using these 3 words. Repeat 3 times.
* Try to concentrate on an object close to you, any object. What do you feel when looking at the object? What thoughts come to your mind when looking at the object?
* Small physical excercise (10 min)
* Small breakfast.
* Nice talk (no complaints, no problematic questions) 10 min. When nobody to talk with, phone or internet conversation oral or written.
* Walk 15 min.

* If you hear voices which are not heard by other people, ask yourself if it is possible to ignore the voices.
Yes
Great! In such a case continue ignoring them.
No
You have to learn to ignore the voices.
This Guide will teach you to ignore the voices.
Remember: even if you cannot stop the voices, the voices cannot stop you to live a normal life.

If you believe in things which other people consider strange, try to keep your strange believes for yourself. Everybody has to make the selection of what can be told to other people and what must be private. Believe me, many people have strange believes. Even much stranger than yours. And they are not considered to be sick. Why? Because they keep their strange believes for themselves. That is the secret.

***

Afternoon
* Think of three different words, any words which just come to your mind at the moment

and make a simple story using these 3 words. Repeat 3 times.
* Try to concentrate on an object close to you, any object. What do you feel when looking at the object? What thoughts come to your mind when looking at the object?
* Dinner and half an hour break (you can sleep).
* Nice talk (no complaints) 15 min. When nobody to talk with, phone or internet conversation oral or written.
* Walk 20 min.
* If you hear voices which are not heard by other people, ask yourself if it is possible to ignore them.

Yes

Great! In such a case continue ignoring them.

No

You have to learn to ignore the voices.
This Guide will teach you to ignore the voices.
Remember: even if you cannot stop the voices, the voices cannot stop you to live a normal life.

If you believe in things which other people consider strange, try to keep your strange believes for yourself. Everybody has to make the selection of what can be told to other people

and what must be private. Believe me, many people have strange believes. Even much stranger than yours. And they are not considered to be sick. Why? Because they keep their strange believes for themselves. That is the secret.

***

Evening

- Think of three different words, any words which just come to your mind at the moment and make a simple story using these 3 words. Repeat 3 times.
- Try to concentrate on an object close to you, any object. What do you feel when looking at the object? What thoughts come to your mind when looking at the object?
- Small supper.
- Nice talk (no complaints) 10 min. When nobody to talk with, phone or internet conversation oral or written.
- Walk 10 min.
- If you hear voices which are not heard by other people, ask yourself if it is possible to ignore them.
Yes

Great! In such a case continue ignoring them.
No
You have to learn to ignore the voices.
This Guide will teach you to ignore the voices.
Remember: even if you cannot stop the voices, the voices cannot stop you to live a normal life.

If you believe in things which other people consider strange, try to keep your strange believes for yourself. Everybody has to make the selection of what can be told to other people and what must be private. Believe me, many people have strange believes. Even much stranger than yours. And they are not considered to be sick. Why? Because they keep their strange believes for themselves. That is the secret.
***

Night
Before sleep
- Take a shower (warm water) 1 min.
- Small physical excercise 3 min.

In Bed
- Repeat STOP (10 times if you hear the voices.
- Think of three different words, any words which just come to your mind at the moment

and make a simple story using these 3 words. Repeat untill you fall asleep.
If you cannot fall asleep
- Think of three different words, any words which just come to your mind at the moment and make a simple story using these 3 words. Repeat untill you fall asleep.

If above does not help
- Stand up and go to the toilet (when possible with as little light as possible)
- Think of three different words, any words which just come to your mind at the moment and make a simple story using these 3 words. Repeat untill you fall asleep.

If above does not help
- Say STOP untill you fall asleep

If above does not help
- Go to the kitchen and have a very small snack.
- Back to the bed think of three different words, any words which just come to your mind at the moment and make a simple story using these 3 words. Repeat untill you fall asleep.
- If above does not help think of three different words, any words which just come to your mind at the moment and make a simple story using these 3 words. Repeat untill you fall asleep.

***

Day 2

Morning

* Say STOP when the voices you hear in your head become too loud to hear your own thoughts.
* If above does not help to stop the voices, just turn your attention away from the voices. The best way to turn your attention away from the voices in your head is by doing one of your favorite occupations. Do not be ashamed of any occupation to turn your attention away from the voices in your head. ALWAYS be busy with your favorite occupation when unsupportable voices come to your head.
* Be careful to keep for yourself these of your believes which are found to be strange by the people.
* CONTROL what you say. Say only things which are not strange for the people. You surely already know which of your believes are found to be strange by the people.
* If you do not know yet which of your believes are found to be strange by the people, OBSERVE how people react on what you say. If you see

that people are ALERTED by your believes, it means your believes are strange. From now on AVOID presenting such believes.

* Think of three different words, any words which just come to your mind at the moment and make a simple story using these 3 words. Repeat 3 times.
* Try to concentrate on an object close to you, any object. What do you feel when looking at the object? What thoughts come to your mind when looking at the object?
* Small physical excercise (10 min)
* Small breakfast.
* Nice talk (no complaints, no problematic questions) 10 min. When nobody to talk with, phone or internet conversation oral or written.
* Walk 15 min.
* If you hear voices which are not heard by other people, ask yourself if it is possible to ignore the voices.

Yes

Great! In such a case continue ignoring them.

No

You have to learn to ignore the voices.
This Guide will teach you to ignore the voices.

Remember: even if you cannot stop the voices, the voices cannot stop you to live a normal life.

If you believe in things which other people consider strange, try to keep your strange believes for yourself. Everybody has to make the selection of what can be told to other people and what must be private. Believe me, many people have strange believes. Even much stranger than yours. And they are not considered to be sick. Why? Because they keep their strange believes for themselves. That is the secret.

***

Afternoon
* Think of three different words, any words which just come to your mind at the moment and make a simple story using these 3 words. Repeat 3 times.
* Try to concentrate on an object close to you, any object. What do you feel when looking at the object? What thoughts come to your mind when looking at the object?
* Dinner and half an hour break (you can sleep).

* Nice talk (no complaints) 15 min. When nobody to talk with, phone or internet conversation oral or written.
* Walk 20 min.
* If you hear voices which are not heard by other people, ask yourself if it is possible to ignore them.

Yes

Great! In such a case continue ignoring them.

No

You have to learn to ignore the voices. This Guide will teach you to ignore the voices. Remember: even if you cannot stop the voices, the voices cannot stop you to live a normal life.

If you believe in things which other people consider strange, try to keep your strange believes for yourself. Everybody has to make the selection of what can be told to other people and what must be private. Believe me, many people have strange believes. Even much stranger than yours. And they are not considered to be sick. Why? Because they keep their strange believes for themselves. That is the secret.

***

Evening

- Think of three different words, any words which just come to your mind at the moment and make a simple story using these 3 words. Repeat 3 times.
- Try to concentrate on an object close to you, any object. What do you feel when looking at the object? What thoughts come to your mind when looking at the object?
- Small supper.
- Nice talk (no complaints) 10 min. When nobody to talk with, phone or internet conversation oral or written.
- Walk 10 min.
- If you hear voices which are not heard by other people, ask yourself if it is possible to ignore them.

Yes

Great! In such a case continue ignoring them.

No

You have to learn to ignore the voices.

This Guide will teach you to ignore the voices.

Remember: even if you cannot stop the voices, the voices cannot stop you to live a normal life.

If you believe in things which other people consider strange, try to keep your strange believes for yourself. Everybody has to make the selection of what can be told to other people and what must be private. Believe me, many people have strange believes. Even much stranger than yours. And they are not considered to be sick. Why? Because they keep their strange believes for themselves. That is the secret.

***

Night
Before sleep
- Take a shower (warm water) 1 min.
- Small physical excercise 3 min.

In Bed
- Repeat STOP (10 times if you hear the voices.
- Think of three different words, any words which just come to your mind at the moment and make a simple story using these 3 words. Repeat untill you fall asleep.

If you cannot fall asleep
- Think of three different words, any words which just come to your mind at the moment and make a simple story using these 3 words. Repeat untill you fall asleep.

If above does not help
- Stand up and go to the toilet (when possible with as little light as possible)
- Think of three different words, any words which just come to your mind at the moment and make a simple story using these 3 words. Repeat untill you fall asleep.

If above does not help
- Say STOP untill you fall asleep

If above does not help
- Go to the kitchen and have a very small snack.
- Back to the bed think of three different words, any words which just come to your mind at the moment and make a simple story using these 3 words. Repeat untill you fall asleep.
- If above does not help think of three different words, any words which just come to your mind at the moment and make a simple story using these 3 words. Repeat untill you fall asleep.

***

Day 3
Morning
* Say STOP when the voices you hear in your head become too loud to hear your own thoughts.

* If above does not help to stop the voices, just turn your attention away from the voices. The best way to turn your attention away from the voices in your head is by doing one of your favorite occupations. Do not be ashamed of any occupation to turn your attention away from the voices in your head. ALWAYS be busy with your favorite occupation when unsupportable voices come to your head.
* Be careful to keep for yourself these of your believes which are found to be strange by the people.
* CONTROL what you say. Say only things which are not strange for the people. You surely already know which of your believes are found to be strange by the people.
* If you do not know yet which of your believes are found to be strange by the people, OBSERVE how people react on what you say. If you see that people are ALERTED by your believes, it means your believes are strange. From now on AVOID presenting such believes.
* Think of three different words, any words which just come to your mind at the moment and make a simple story using these 3 words. Repeat 3 times.

* Try to concentrate on an object close to you, any object. What do you feel when looking at the object? What thoughts come to your mind when looking at the object?
* Small physical excercise (10 min)
* Small breakfast.
* Nice talk (no complaints, no problematic questions) 10 min. When nobody to talk with, phone or internet conversation oral or written.
* Walk 15 min.
* If you hear voices which are not heard by other people, ask yourself if it is possible to ignore the voices.

Yes

Great! In such a case continue ignoring them.

No

You have to learn to ignore the voices.
This Guide will teach you to ignore the voices. Remember: even if you cannot stop the voices, the voices cannot stop you to live a normal life.

If you believe in things which other people consider strange, try to keep your strange believes for yourself. Everybody has to make the selection of what can be told to other people and what must be private. Believe me, many people have strange believes. Even much stranger than yours. And they are not considered to be sick. Why? Because they keep their strange believes for themselves. That is the secret.

***

Afternoon
* Think of three different words, any words which just come to your mind at the moment and make a simple story using these 3 words. Repeat 3 times.
* Try to concentrate on an object close to you, any object. What do you feel when looking at the object? What thoughts come to your mind when looking at the object?
* Dinner and half an hour break (you can sleep).
* Nice talk (no complaints) 15 min. When nobody to talk with, phone or internet conversation oral or written.
* Walk 20 min.
* If you hear voices which are not heard by other people, ask yourself if it is possible to ignore them.
Yes
Great! In such a case continue ignoring them.

No

You have to learn to ignore the voices.
This Guide will teach you to ignore the voices.
Remember: even if you cannot stop the voices, the voices cannot stop you to live a normal life.

If you believe in things which other people consider strange, try to keep your strange believes for yourself. Everybody has to make the selection of what can be told to other people and what must be private. Believe me, many people have strange believes. Even much stranger than yours. And they are not considered to be sick. Why? Because they keep their strange believes for themselves. That is the secret.

***

Evening

- Think of three different words, any words which just come to your mind at the moment and make a simple story using these 3 words. Repeat 3 times.
- Try to concentrate on an object close to you, any object. What do you feel when looking at

the object? What thoughts come to your mind when looking at the object?
- Small supper.
- Nice talk (no complaints) 10 min. When nobody to talk with, phone or internet conversation oral or written.
- Walk 10 min.
- If you hear voices which are not heard by other people, ask yourself if it is possible to ignore them.

Yes

Great! In such a case continue ignoring them.

No

You have to learn to ignore the voices.
This Guide will teach you to ignore the voices. Remember: even if you cannot stop the voices, the voices cannot stop you to live a normal life.

If you believe in things which other people consider strange, try to keep your strange believes for yourself. Everybody has to make the selection of what can be told to other people and what must be private. Believe me, many people have strange believes. Even much stranger than yours. And they are not considered to be sick. Why? Because they keep

their strange believes for themselves. That is the secret.

***

Night

Before sleep
- Take a shower (warm water) 1 min.
- Small physical excercise 3 min.

In Bed
- Repeat STOP (10 times if you hear the voices.
- Think of three different words, any words which just come to your mind at the moment and make a simple story using these 3 words. Repeat untill you fall asleep.

If you cannot fall asleep
- Think of three different words, any words which just come to your mind at the moment and make a simple story using these 3 words. Repeat untill you fall asleep.

If above does not help
- Stand up and go to the toilet (when possible with as little light as possible)
- Think of three different words, any words which just come to your mind at the moment and make a simple story using these 3 words. Repeat untill you fall asleep.

If above does not help

- Say STOP untill you fall asleep

If above does not help
- Go to the kitchen and have a very small snack.
- Back to the bed think of three different words, any words which just come to your mind at the moment and make a simple story using these 3 words. Repeat untill you fall asleep.
- If above does not help think of three different words, any words which just come to your mind at the moment and make a simple story using these 3 words. Repeat untill you fall asleep.

***

Day 4

Morning

* Say STOP when the voices you hear in your head become too loud to hear your own thoughts.
* If above does not help to stop the voices, just turn your attention away from the voices. The best way to turn your attention away from the voices in your head is by doing one of your favorite occupations. Do not be ashamed of any occupation to turn your attention away from the voices in your head. ALWAYS be busy with your

favorite occupation when unsupportable voices come to your head.
* Be careful to keep for yourself these of your believes which are found to be strange by the people.
* CONTROL what you say. Say only things which are not strange for the people. You surely already know which of your believes are found to be strange by the people.
* If you do not know yet which of your believes are found to be strange by the people, OBSERVE how people react on what you say. If you see that people are ALERTED by your believes, it means your believes are strange. From now on AVOID presenting such believes.
* Think of three different words, any words which just come to your mind at the moment and make a simple story using these 3 words. Repeat 3 times.
* Try to concentrate on an object close to you, any object. What do you feel when looking at the object? What thoughts come to your mind when looking at the object?
* Small physical excercise (10 min)
* Small breakfast.

* Nice talk (no complaints, no problematic questions) 10 min. When nobody to talk with, phone or internet conversation oral or written.
* Walk 15 min.
* If you hear voices which are not heard by other people, ask yourself if it is possible to ignore the voices.

Yes

Great! In such a case continue ignoring them.

No

You have to learn to ignore the voices.
This Guide will teach you to ignore the voices.
Remember: even if you cannot stop the voices, the voices cannot stop you to live a normal life.

If you believe in things which other people consider strange, try to keep your strange believes for yourself. Everybody has to make the selection of what can be told to other people and what must be private. Believe me, many people have strange believes. Even much stranger than yours. And they are not considered to be sick. Why? Because they keep their strange believes for themselves. That is the secret.

***

Afternoon

* Think of three different words, any words which just come to your mind at the moment and make a simple story using these 3 words. Repeat 3 times.
* Try to concentrate on an object close to you, any object. What do you feel when looking at the object? What thoughts come to your mind when looking at the object?
* Dinner and half an hour break (you can sleep).
* Nice talk (no complaints) 15 min. When nobody to talk with, phone or internet conversation oral or written.
* Walk 20 min.
* If you hear voices which are not heard by other people, ask yourself if it is possible to ignore them.

Yes

Great! In such a case continue ignoring them.

No

You have to learn to ignore the voices.

This Guide will teach you to ignore the voices.

Remember: even if you cannot stop the voices, the voices cannot stop you to live a normal life.

If you believe in things which other people consider strange, try to keep your strange believes for yourself. Everybody has to make the selection of what can be told to other people and what must be private. Believe me, many people have strange believes. Even much stranger than yours. And they are not considered to be sick. Why? Because they keep their strange believes for themselves. That is the secret.

***

Evening

- Think of three different words, any words which just come to your mind at the moment and make a simple story using these 3 words. Repeat 3 times.
- Try to concentrate on an object close to you, any object. What do you feel when looking at the object? What thoughts come to your mind when looking at the object?
- Small supper.
- Nice talk (no complaints) 10 min. When nobody to talk with, phone or internet conversation oral or written.
- Walk 10 min.

- If you hear voices which are not heard by other people, ask yourself if it is possible to ignore them.

Yes

Great! In such a case continue ignoring them.

No

You have to learn to ignore the voices.
This Guide will teach you to ignore the voices. Remember: even if you cannot stop the voices, the voices cannot stop you to live a normal life.

If you believe in things which other people consider strange, try to keep your strange believes for yourself. Everybody has to make the selection of what can be told to other people and what must be private. Believe me, many people have strange believes. Even much stranger than yours. And they are not considered to be sick. Why? Because they keep their strange believes for themselves. That is the secret.

***

Night

Before sleep
- Take a shower (warm water) 1 min.
- Small physical excercise 3 min.

In Bed
- Repeat STOP (10 times if you hear the voices.
- Think of three different words, any words which just come to your mind at the moment and make a simple story using these 3 words. Repeat untill you fall asleep.

If you cannot fall asleep
- Think of three different words, any words which just come to your mind at the moment and make a simple story using these 3 words. Repeat untill you fall asleep.

If above does not help
- Stand up and go to the toilet (when possible with as little light as possible)
- Think of three different words, any words which just come to your mind at the moment and make a simple story using these 3 words. Repeat untill you fall asleep.

If above does not help
- Say STOP untill you fall asleep

If above does not help
- Go to the kitchen and have a very small snack.
- Back to the bed think of three different words, any words which just come to your mind at the moment and make a simple story using these 3 words. Repeat untill you fall asleep.

- If above does not help think of three different words, any words which just come to your mind at the moment and make a simple story using these 3 words. Repeat untill you fall asleep.

***

Day 5

Morning

* Say STOP when the voices you hear in your head become too loud to hear your own thoughts.
* If above does not help to stop the voices, just turn your attention away from the voices. The best way to turn your attention away from the voices in your head is by doing one of your favorite occupations. Do not be ashamed of any occupation to turn your attention away from the voices in your head. ALWAYS be busy with your favorite occupation when unsupportable voices come to your head.
* Be careful to keep for yourself these of your believes which are found to be strange by the people.
* CONTROL what you say. Say only things which are not strange for the people. You surely

already know which of your believes are found to be strange by the people.
* If you do not know yet which of your believes are found to be strange by the people, OBSERVE how people react on what you say. If you see that people are ALERTED by your believes, it means your believes are strange. From now on AVOID presenting such believes.
* Think of three different words, any words which just come to your mind at the moment and make a simple story using these 3 words. Repeat 3 times.
* Try to concentrate on an object close to you, any object. What do you feel when looking at the object? What thoughts come to your mind when looking at the object?
* Small physical excercise (10 min)
* Small breakfast.
* Nice talk (no complaints, no problematic questions) 10 min. When nobody to talk with, phone or internet conversation oral or written.
* Walk 15 min.
* If you hear voices which are not heard by other people, ask yourself if it is possible to ignore the voices.
Yes

Great! In such a case continue ignoring them.
No
You have to learn to ignore the voices.
This Guide will teach you to ignore the voices.
Remember: even if you cannot stop the voices, the voices cannot stop you to live a normal life.

If you believe in things which other people consider strange, try to keep your strange believes for yourself. Everybody has to make the selection of what can be told to other people and what must be private. Believe me, many people have strange believes. Even much stranger than yours. And they are not considered to be sick. Why? Because they keep their strange believes for themselves. That is the secret.

***

Afternoon
* Think of three different words, any words which just come to your mind at the moment and make a simple story using these 3 words. Repeat 3 times.
* Try to concentrate on an object close to you, any object. What do you feel when looking at

the object? What thoughts come to your mind when looking at the object?
* Dinner and half an hour break (you can sleep).
* Nice talk (no complaints) 15 min. When nobody to talk with, phone or internet conversation oral or written.
* Walk 20 min.
* If you hear voices which are not heard by other people, ask yourself if it is possible to ignore them.

Yes

Great! In such a case continue ignoring them.

No

You have to learn to ignore the voices.
This Guide will teach you to ignore the voices.
Remember: even if you cannot stop the voices, the voices cannot stop you to live a normal life.

If you believe in things which other people consider strange, try to keep your strange believes for yourself. Everybody has to make the selection of what can be told to other people and what must be private. Believe me, many people have strange believes. Even much stranger than yours. And they are not considered to be sick. Why? Because they keep

their strange believes for themselves. That is the secret.

***

Evening

- Think of three different words, any words which just come to your mind at the moment and make a simple story using these 3 words. Repeat 3 times.
- Try to concentrate on an object close to you, any object. What do you feel when looking at the object? What thoughts come to your mind when looking at the object?
- Small supper.
- Nice talk (no complaints) 10 min. When nobody to talk with, phone or internet conversation oral or written.
- Walk 10 min.
- If you hear voices which are not heard by other people, ask yourself if it is possible to ignore them.

Yes

Great! In such a case continue ignoring them.

No

You have to learn to ignore the voices.
This Guide will teach you to ignore the voices.

Remember: even if you cannot stop the voices, the voices cannot stop you to live a normal life.

If you believe in things which other people consider strange, try to keep your strange believes for yourself. Everybody has to make the selection of what can be told to other people and what must be private. Believe me, many people have strange believes. Even much stranger than yours. And they are not considered to be sick. Why? Because they keep their strange believes for themselves. That is the secret.

***

Night
Before sleep
- Take a shower (warm water) 1 min.
- Small physical excercise 3 min.

In Bed
- Repeat STOP (10 times if you hear the voices.
- Think of three different words, any words which just come to your mind at the moment and make a simple story using these 3 words. Repeat untill you fall asleep.

If you cannot fall asleep

- Think of three different words, any words which just come to your mind at the moment and make a simple story using these 3 words. Repeat untill you fall asleep.

If above does not help
- Stand up and go to the toilet (when possible with as little light as possible)
- Think of three different words, any words which just come to your mind at the moment and make a simple story using these 3 words. Repeat untill you fall asleep.

If above does not help
- Say STOP untill you fall asleep

If above does not help
- Go to the kitchen and have a very small snack.
- Back to the bed think of three different words, any words which just come to your mind at the moment and make a simple story using these 3 words. Repeat untill you fall asleep.
- If above does not help think of three different words, any words which just come to your mind at the moment and make a simple story using these 3 words. Repeat untill you fall asleep.

***

Day 6

Morning
* Say STOP when the voices you hear in your head become too loud to hear your own thoughts.
* If above does not help to stop the voices, just turn your attention away from the voices. The best way to turn your attention away from the voices in your head is by doing one of your favorite occupations. Do not be ashamed of any occupation to turn your attention away from the voices in your head. ALWAYS be busy with your favorite occupation when unsupportable voices come to your head.
* Be careful to keep for yourself these of your believes which are found to be strange by the people.
* CONTROL what you say. Say only things which are not strange for the people. You surely already know which of your believes are found to be strange by the people.
* If you do not know yet which of your believes are found to be strange by the people, OBSERVE how people react on what you say. If you see that people are ALERTED by your believes, it means your believes are strange. From now on AVOID presenting such believes.

* Think of three different words, any words which just come to your mind at the moment and make a simple story using these 3 words. Repeat 3 times.
* Try to concentrate on an object close to you, any object. What do you feel when looking at the object? What thoughts come to your mind when looking at the object?
* Small physical excercise (10 min)
* Small breakfast.
* Nice talk (no complaints, no problematic questions) 10 min. When nobody to talk with, phone or internet conversation oral or written.
* Walk 15 min.
* If you hear voices which are not heard by other people, ask yourself if it is possible to ignore the voices.

Yes

Great! In such a case continue ignoring them.

No

You have to learn to ignore the voices.

This Guide will teach you to ignore the voices. Remember: even if you cannot stop the voices, the voices cannot stop you to live a normal life.

If you believe in things which other people consider strange, try to keep your strange believes for yourself. Everybody has to make the selection of what can be told to other people and what must be private. Believe me, many people have strange believes. Even much stranger than yours. And they are not considered to be sick. Why? Because they keep their strange believes for themselves. That is the secret.

***

Afternoon
* Think of three different words, any words which just come to your mind at the moment and make a simple story using these 3 words. Repeat 3 times.
* Try to concentrate on an object close to you, any object. What do you feel when looking at the object? What thoughts come to your mind when looking at the object?
* Dinner and half an hour break (you can sleep).
* Nice talk (no complaints) 15 min. When nobody to talk with, phone or internet conversation oral or written.
* Walk 20 min.

* If you hear voices which are not heard by other people, ask yourself if it is possible to ignore them.
Yes
Great! In such a case continue ignoring them.
No
You have to learn to ignore the voices.
This Guide will teach you to ignore the voices.
Remember: even if you cannot stop the voices, the voices cannot stop you to live a normal life.

If you believe in things which other people consider strange, try to keep your strange believes for yourself. Everybody has to make the selection of what can be told to other people and what must be private. Believe me, many people have strange believes. Even much stranger than yours. And they are not considered to be sick. Why? Because they keep their strange believes for themselves. That is the secret.
***
Evening

• Think of three different words, any words which just come to your mind at the moment

and make a simple story using these 3 words. Repeat 3 times.
- Try to concentrate on an object close to you, any object. What do you feel when looking at the object? What thoughts come to your mind when looking at the object?
- Small supper.
- Nice talk (no complaints) 10 min. When nobody to talk with, phone or internet conversation oral or written.
- Walk 10 min.
- If you hear voices which are not heard by other people, ask yourself if it is possible to ignore them.

Yes

Great! In such a case continue ignoring them.

No

You have to learn to ignore the voices.
This Guide will teach you to ignore the voices.
Remember: even if you cannot stop the voices, the voices cannot stop you to live a normal life.

If you believe in things which other people consider strange, try to keep your strange believes for yourself. Everybody has to make the selection of what can be told to other people

and what must be private. Believe me, many people have strange believes. Even much stranger than yours. And they are not considered to be sick. Why? Because they keep their strange believes for themselves. That is the secret.

***

Night

Before sleep
- Take a shower (warm water) 1 min.
- Small physical excercise 3 min.

In Bed
- Repeat STOP (10 times if you hear the voices.
- Think of three different words, any words which just come to your mind at the moment and make a simple story using these 3 words. Repeat untill you fall asleep.

If you cannot fall asleep
- Think of three different words, any words which just come to your mind at the moment and make a simple story using these 3 words. Repeat untill you fall asleep.

If above does not help
- Stand up and go to the toilet (when possible with as little light as possible)

- Think of three different words, any words which just come to your mind at the moment and make a simple story using these 3 words. Repeat untill you fall asleep.

If above does not help
- Say STOP untill you fall asleep

If above does not help
- Go to the kitchen and have a very small snack.
- Back to the bed think of three different words, any words which just come to your mind at the moment and make a simple story using these 3 words. Repeat untill you fall asleep.
- If above does not help think of three different words, any words which just come to your mind at the moment and make a simple story using these 3 words. Repeat untill you fall asleep.

***

Day 7

Morning

* Say STOP when the voices you hear in your head become too loud to hear your own thoughts.

* If above does not help to stop the voices, just turn your attention away from the voices. The best way to turn your attention away from the

voices in your head is by doing one of your favorite occupations. Do not be ashamed of any occupation to turn your attention away from the voices in your head. ALWAYS be busy with your favorite occupation when unsupportable voices come to your head.

* Be careful to keep for yourself these of your believes which are found to be strange by the people.
* CONTROL what you say. Say only things which are not strange for the people. You surely already know which of your believes are found to be strange by the people.
* If you do not know yet which of your believes are found to be strange by the people, OBSERVE how people react on what you say. If you see that people are ALERTED by your believes, it means your believes are strange. From now on AVOID presenting such believes.
* Think of three different words, any words which just come to your mind at the moment and make a simple story using these 3 words. Repeat 3 times.
* Try to concentrate on an object close to you, any object. What do you feel when looking at

the object? What thoughts come to your mind when looking at the object?
* Small physical excercise (10 min)
* Small breakfast.
* Nice talk (no complaints, no problematic questions) 10 min. When nobody to talk with, phone or internet conversation oral or written.
* Walk 15 min.
* If you hear voices which are not heard by other people, ask yourself if it is possible to ignore the voices.

Yes

Great! In such a case continue ignoring them.

No

You have to learn to ignore the voices.
This Guide will teach you to ignore the voices.
Remember: even if you cannot stop the voices, the voices cannot stop you to live a normal life.

If you believe in things which other people consider strange, try to keep your strange believes for yourself. Everybody has to make the selection of what can be told to other people and what must be private. Believe me, many people have strange believes. Even much stranger than yours. And they are not

considered to be sick. Why? Because they keep their strange believes for themselves. That is the secret.

***

Afternoon
* Think of three different words, any words which just come to your mind at the moment and make a simple story using these 3 words. Repeat 3 times.
* Try to concentrate on an object close to you, any object. What do you feel when looking at the object? What thoughts come to your mind when looking at the object?
* Dinner and half an hour break (you can sleep).
* Nice talk (no complaints) 15 min. When nobody to talk with, phone or internet conversation oral or written.
* Walk 20 min.
* If you hear voices which are not heard by other people, ask yourself if it is possible to ignore them.
Yes
Great! In such a case continue ignoring them.
No
You have to learn to ignore the voices.

This Guide will teach you to ignore the voices. Remember: even if you cannot stop the voices, the voices cannot stop you to live a normal life.

If you believe in things which other people consider strange, try to keep your strange believes for yourself. Everybody has to make the selection of what can be told to other people and what must be private. Believe me, many people have strange believes. Even much stranger than yours. And they are not considered to be sick. Why? Because they keep their strange believes for themselves. That is the secret.

***

Evening

- Think of three different words, any words which just come to your mind at the moment and make a simple story using these 3 words. Repeat 3 times.
- Try to concentrate on an object close to you, any object. What do you feel when looking at the object? What thoughts come to your mind when looking at the object?
- Small supper.

- Nice talk (no complaints) 10 min. When nobody to talk with, phone or internet conversation oral or written.
- Walk 10 min.
- If you hear voices which are not heard by other people, ask yourself if it is possible to ignore them.

Yes

Great! In such a case continue ignoring them.

No

You have to learn to ignore the voices.
This Guide will teach you to ignore the voices.
Remember: even if you cannot stop the voices, the voices cannot stop you to live a normal life.

If you believe in things which other people consider strange, try to keep your strange believes for yourself. Everybody has to make the selection of what can be told to other people and what must be private. Believe me, many people have strange believes. Even much stranger than yours. And they are not considered to be sick. Why? Because they keep their strange believes for themselves. That is the secret.

***

Night

Before sleep
- Take a shower (warm water) 1 min.
- Small physical excercise 3 min.

In Bed
- Repeat STOP (10 times if you hear the voices.
- Think of three different words, any words which just come to your mind at the moment and make a simple story using these 3 words. Repeat untill you fall asleep.

If you cannot fall asleep
- Think of three different words, any words which just come to your mind at the moment and make a simple story using these 3 words. Repeat untill you fall asleep.

If above does not help
- Stand up and go to the toilet (when possible with as little light as possible)
- Think of three different words, any words which just come to your mind at the moment and make a simple story using these 3 words. Repeat untill you fall asleep.

If above does not help
- Say STOP untill you fall asleep

If above does not help
- Go to the kitchen and have a very small snack.

- Back to the bed think of three different words, any words which just come to your mind at the moment and make a simple story using these 3 words. Repeat untill you fall asleep.
- If above does not help think of three different words, any words which just come to your mind at the moment and make a simple story using these 3 words. Repeat untill you fall asleep.

***

Week Four

***

***

Day 1

Morning

* Say STOP when the voices you hear in your head become too loud to hear your own thoughts.
* If above does not help to stop the voices, just turn your attention away from the voices. The best way to turn your attention away from the voices in your head is by doing one of your favorite occupations. Do not be ashamed of any occupation to turn your attention away from the voices in your head. ALWAYS be busy with your

favorite occupation when unsupportable voices come to your head.
* Be careful to keep for yourself these of your believes which are found to be strange by the people.
* CONTROL what you say. Say only things which are not strange for the people. You surely already know which of your believes are found to be strange by the people.
* If you do not know yet which of your believes are found to be strange by the people, OBSERVE how people react on what you say. If you see that people are ALERTED by your believes, it means your believes are strange. From now on AVOID presenting such believes.
* Think of three different words, any words which just come to your mind at the moment and make a simple story using these 3 words. Repeat 3 times.
* Try to concentrate on an object close to you, any object. What do you feel when looking at the object? What thoughts come to your mind when looking at the object?
* Small physical excercise (10 min)
* Small breakfast.

* Nice talk (no complaints, no problematic questions) 10 min. When nobody to talk with, phone or internet conversation oral or written.
* Walk 15 min.
* If you hear voices which are not heard by other people, ask yourself if it is possible to ignore the voices.

Yes

Great! In such a case continue ignoring them.

No

You have to learn to ignore the voices.
This Guide will teach you to ignore the voices.
Remember: even if you cannot stop the voices, the voices cannot stop you to live a normal life.

If you believe in things which other people consider strange, try to keep your strange believes for yourself. Everybody has to make the selection of what can be told to other people and what must be private. Believe me, many people have strange believes. Even much stranger than yours. And they are not considered to be sick. Why? Because they keep their strange believes for themselves. That is the secret.

***

Afternoon

* Think of three different words, any words which just come to your mind at the moment and make a simple story using these 3 words. Repeat 3 times.
* Try to concentrate on an object close to you, any object. What do you feel when looking at the object? What thoughts come to your mind when looking at the object?
* Dinner and half an hour break (you can sleep).
* Nice talk (no complaints) 15 min. When nobody to talk with, phone or internet conversation oral or written.
* Walk 20 min.
* If you hear voices which are not heard by other people, ask yourself if it is possible to ignore them.

Yes

Great! In such a case continue ignoring them.

No

You have to learn to ignore the voices.

This Guide will teach you to ignore the voices.

Remember: even if you cannot stop the voices, the voices cannot stop you to live a normal life.

If you believe in things which other people consider strange, try to keep your strange believes for yourself. Everybody has to make the selection of what can be told to other people and what must be private. Believe me, many people have strange believes. Even much stranger than yours. And they are not considered to be sick. Why? Because they keep their strange believes for themselves. That is the secret.

***

Evening

- Think of three different words, any words which just come to your mind at the moment and make a simple story using these 3 words. Repeat 3 times.
- Try to concentrate on an object close to you, any object. What do you feel when looking at the object? What thoughts come to your mind when looking at the object?
- Small supper.
- Nice talk (no complaints) 10 min. When nobody to talk with, phone or internet conversation oral or written.
- Walk 10 min.

- If you hear voices which are not heard by other people, ask yourself if it is possible to ignore them.

Yes
Great! In such a case continue ignoring them.
No
You have to learn to ignore the voices.
This Guide will teach you to ignore the voices.
Remember: even if you cannot stop the voices, the voices cannot stop you to live a normal life.

If you believe in things which other people consider strange, try to keep your strange believes for yourself. Everybody has to make the selection of what can be told to other people and what must be private. Believe me, many people have strange believes. Even much stranger than yours. And they are not considered to be sick. Why? Because they keep their strange believes for themselves. That is the secret.

***

Night
Before sleep
- Take a shower (warm water) 1 min.
- Small physical excercise 3 min.

In Bed
- Repeat STOP (10 times if you hear the voices.
- Think of three different words, any words which just come to your mind at the moment and make a simple story using these 3 words. Repeat untill you fall asleep.

If you cannot fall asleep
- Think of three different words, any words which just come to your mind at the moment and make a simple story using these 3 words. Repeat untill you fall asleep.

If above does not help
- Stand up and go to the toilet (when possible with as little light as possible)
- Think of three different words, any words which just come to your mind at the moment and make a simple story using these 3 words. Repeat untill you fall asleep.

If above does not help
- Say STOP untill you fall asleep

If above does not help
- Go to the kitchen and have a very small snack.
- Back to the bed think of three different words, any words which just come to your mind at the moment and make a simple story using these 3 words. Repeat untill you fall asleep.

- If above does not help think of three different words, any words which just come to your mind at the moment and make a simple story using these 3 words. Repeat untill you fall asleep.

***

Day 2

Morning

* Say STOP when the voices you hear in your head become too loud to hear your own thoughts.
* If above does not help to stop the voices, just turn your attention away from the voices. The best way to turn your attention away from the voices in your head is by doing one of your favorite occupations. Do not be ashamed of any occupation to turn your attention away from the voices in your head. ALWAYS be busy with your favorite occupation when unsupportable voices come to your head.
* Be careful to keep for yourself these of your believes which are found to be strange by the people.
* CONTROL what you say. Say only things which are not strange for the people. You surely

already know which of your believes are found to be strange by the people.
* If you do not know yet which of your believes are found to be strange by the people, OBSERVE how people react on what you say. If you see that people are ALERTED by your believes, it means your believes are strange. From now on AVOID presenting such believes.
* Think of three different words, any words which just come to your mind at the moment and make a simple story using these 3 words. Repeat 3 times.
* Try to concentrate on an object close to you, any object. What do you feel when looking at the object? What thoughts come to your mind when looking at the object?
* Small physical excercise (10 min)
* Small breakfast.
* Nice talk (no complaints, no problematic questions) 10 min. When nobody to talk with, phone or internet conversation oral or written.
* Walk 15 min.
* If you hear voices which are not heard by other people, ask yourself if it is possible to ignore the voices.
Yes

Great! In such a case continue ignoring them.
No
You have to learn to ignore the voices.
This Guide will teach you to ignore the voices.
Remember: even if you cannot stop the voices, the voices cannot stop you to live a normal life.

If you believe in things which other people consider strange, try to keep your strange believes for yourself. Everybody has to make the selection of what can be told to other people and what must be private. Believe me, many people have strange believes. Even much stranger than yours. And they are not considered to be sick. Why? Because they keep their strange believes for themselves. That is the secret.

***

Afternoon
* Think of three different words, any words which just come to your mind at the moment and make a simple story using these 3 words. Repeat 3 times.
* Try to concentrate on an object close to you, any object. What do you feel when looking at

the object? What thoughts come to your mind when looking at the object?
* Dinner and half an hour break (you can sleep).
* Nice talk (no complaints) 15 min. When nobody to talk with, phone or internet conversation oral or written.
* Walk 20 min.
* If you hear voices which are not heard by other people, ask yourself if it is possible to ignore them.
Yes
Great! In such a case continue ignoring them.
No
You have to learn to ignore the voices.
This Guide will teach you to ignore the voices.
Remember: even if you cannot stop the voices, the voices cannot stop you to live a normal life.

If you believe in things which other people consider strange, try to keep your strange believes for yourself. Everybody has to make the selection of what can be told to other people and what must be private. Believe me, many people have strange believes. Even much stranger than yours. And they are not considered to be sick. Why? Because they keep

their strange believes for themselves. That is the secret.

***

Evening

- Think of three different words, any words which just come to your mind at the moment and make a simple story using these 3 words. Repeat 3 times.
- Try to concentrate on an object close to you, any object. What do you feel when looking at the object? What thoughts come to your mind when looking at the object?
- Small supper.
- Nice talk (no complaints) 10 min. When nobody to talk with, phone or internet conversation oral or written.
- Walk 10 min.
- If you hear voices which are not heard by other people, ask yourself if it is possible to ignore them.

Yes

Great! In such a case continue ignoring them.

No

You have to learn to ignore the voices.

This Guide will teach you to ignore the voices.

Remember: even if you cannot stop the voices, the voices cannot stop you to live a normal life.

If you believe in things which other people consider strange, try to keep your strange believes for yourself. Everybody has to make the selection of what can be told to other people and what must be private. Believe me, many people have strange believes. Even much stranger than yours. And they are not considered to be sick. Why? Because they keep their strange believes for themselves. That is the secret.
***

Night
Before sleep
- Take a shower (warm water) 1 min.
- Small physical excercise 3 min.

In Bed
- Repeat STOP (10 times if you hear the voices.
- Think of three different words, any words which just come to your mind at the moment and make a simple story using these 3 words. Repeat untill you fall asleep.

If you cannot fall asleep

- Think of three different words, any words which just come to your mind at the moment and make a simple story using these 3 words. Repeat untill you fall asleep.

If above does not help
- Stand up and go to the toilet (when possible with as little light as possible)
- Think of three different words, any words which just come to your mind at the moment and make a simple story using these 3 words. Repeat untill you fall asleep.

If above does not help
- Say STOP untill you fall asleep

If above does not help
- Go to the kitchen and have a very small snack.
- Back to the bed think of three different words, any words which just come to your mind at the moment and make a simple story using these 3 words. Repeat untill you fall asleep.
- If above does not help think of three different words, any words which just come to your mind at the moment and make a simple story using these 3 words. Repeat untill you fall asleep.

***

Day 3

Morning
* Say STOP when the voices you hear in your head become too loud to hear your own thoughts.
* If above does not help to stop the voices, just turn your attention away from the voices. The best way to turn your attention away from the voices in your head is by doing one of your favorite occupations. Do not be ashamed of any occupation to turn your attention away from the voices in your head. ALWAYS be busy with your favorite occupation when unsupportable voices come to your head.
* Be careful to keep for yourself these of your believes which are found to be strange by the people.
* CONTROL what you say. Say only things which are not strange for the people. You surely already know which of your believes are found to be strange by the people.
* If you do not know yet which of your believes are found to be strange by the people, OBSERVE how people react on what you say. If you see that people are ALERTED by your believes, it means your believes are strange. From now on AVOID presenting such believes.

* Think of three different words, any words which just come to your mind at the moment and make a simple story using these 3 words. Repeat 3 times.
* Try to concentrate on an object close to you, any object. What do you feel when looking at the object? What thoughts come to your mind when looking at the object?
* Small physical excercise (10 min)
* Small breakfast.
* Nice talk (no complaints, no problematic questions) 10 min. When nobody to talk with, phone or internet conversation oral or written.
* Walk 15 min.
* If you hear voices which are not heard by other people, ask yourself if it is possible to ignore the voices.

Yes

Great! In such a case continue ignoring them.

No

You have to learn to ignore the voices.
This Guide will teach you to ignore the voices.
Remember: even if you cannot stop the voices, the voices cannot stop you to live a normal life.

If you believe in things which other people consider strange, try to keep your strange believes for yourself. Everybody has to make the selection of what can be told to other people and what must be private. Believe me, many people have strange believes. Even much stranger than yours. And they are not considered to be sick. Why? Because they keep their strange believes for themselves. That is the secret.

***

Afternoon
* Think of three different words, any words which just come to your mind at the moment and make a simple story using these 3 words. Repeat 3 times.
* Try to concentrate on an object close to you, any object. What do you feel when looking at the object? What thoughts come to your mind when looking at the object?
* Dinner and half an hour break (you can sleep).
* Nice talk (no complaints) 15 min. When nobody to talk with, phone or internet conversation oral or written.
* Walk 20 min.

* If you hear voices which are not heard by other people, ask yourself if it is possible to ignore them.
Yes
Great! In such a case continue ignoring them.
No
You have to learn to ignore the voices.
This Guide will teach you to ignore the voices.
Remember: even if you cannot stop the voices, the voices cannot stop you to live a normal life.

If you believe in things which other people consider strange, try to keep your strange believes for yourself. Everybody has to make the selection of what can be told to other people and what must be private. Believe me, many people have strange believes. Even much stranger than yours. And they are not considered to be sick. Why? Because they keep their strange believes for themselves. That is the secret.

***

Evening

- Think of three different words, any words which just come to your mind at the moment

and make a simple story using these 3 words. Repeat 3 times.
- Try to concentrate on an object close to you, any object. What do you feel when looking at the object? What thoughts come to your mind when looking at the object?
- Small supper.
- Nice talk (no complaints) 10 min. When nobody to talk with, phone or internet conversation oral or written.
- Walk 10 min.
- If you hear voices which are not heard by other people, ask yourself if it is possible to ignore them.

Yes

Great! In such a case continue ignoring them.

No

You have to learn to ignore the voices.
This Guide will teach you to ignore the voices.
Remember: even if you cannot stop the voices, the voices cannot stop you to live a normal life.

If you believe in things which other people consider strange, try to keep your strange believes for yourself. Everybody has to make the selection of what can be told to other people

and what must be private. Believe me, many people have strange believes. Even much stranger than yours. And they are not considered to be sick. Why? Because they keep their strange believes for themselves. That is the secret.

***

Night

Before sleep
- Take a shower (warm water) 1 min.
- Small physical excercise 3 min.

In Bed
- Repeat STOP (10 times if you hear the voices.
- Think of three different words, any words which just come to your mind at the moment and make a simple story using these 3 words. Repeat untill you fall asleep.

If you cannot fall asleep
- Think of three different words, any words which just come to your mind at the moment and make a simple story using these 3 words. Repeat untill you fall asleep.

If above does not help
- Stand up and go to the toilet (when possible with as little light as possible)

- Think of three different words, any words which just come to your mind at the moment and make a simple story using these 3 words. Repeat untill you fall asleep.

If above does not help
- Say STOP untill you fall asleep

If above does not help
- Go to the kitchen and have a very small snack.
- Back to the bed think of three different words, any words which just come to your mind at the moment and make a simple story using these 3 words. Repeat untill you fall asleep.
- If above does not help think of three different words, any words which just come to your mind at the moment and make a simple story using these 3 words. Repeat untill you fall asleep.

***

Day 4

Morning

* Say STOP when the voices you hear in your head become too loud to hear your own thoughts.

* If above does not help to stop the voices, just turn your attention away from the voices. The best way to turn your attention away from the

voices in your head is by doing one of your favorite occupations. Do not be ashamed of any occupation to turn your attention away from the voices in your head. ALWAYS be busy with your favorite occupation when unsupportable voices come to your head.

* Be careful to keep for yourself these of your believes which are found to be strange by the people.
* CONTROL what you say. Say only things which are not strange for the people. You surely already know which of your believes are found to be strange by the people.
* If you do not know yet which of your believes are found to be strange by the people, OBSERVE how people react on what you say. If you see that people are ALERTED by your believes, it means your believes are strange. From now on AVOID presenting such believes.
* Think of three different words, any words which just come to your mind at the moment and make a simple story using these 3 words. Repeat 3 times.
* Try to concentrate on an object close to you, any object. What do you feel when looking at

the object? What thoughts come to your mind when looking at the object?
* Small physical excercise (10 min)
* Small breakfast.
* Nice talk (no complaints, no problematic questions) 10 min. When nobody to talk with, phone or internet conversation oral or written.
* Walk 15 min.
* If you hear voices which are not heard by other people, ask yourself if it is possible to ignore the voices.

Yes

Great! In such a case continue ignoring them.

No

You have to learn to ignore the voices.
This Guide will teach you to ignore the voices.
Remember: even if you cannot stop the voices, the voices cannot stop you to live a normal life.

If you believe in things which other people consider strange, try to keep your strange believes for yourself. Everybody has to make the selection of what can be told to other people and what must be private. Believe me, many people have strange believes. Even much stranger than yours. And they are not

considered to be sick. Why? Because they keep their strange believes for themselves. That is the secret.

***

Afternoon
* Think of three different words, any words which just come to your mind at the moment and make a simple story using these 3 words. Repeat 3 times.
* Try to concentrate on an object close to you, any object. What do you feel when looking at the object? What thoughts come to your mind when looking at the object?
* Dinner and half an hour break (you can sleep).
* Nice talk (no complaints) 15 min. When nobody to talk with, phone or internet conversation oral or written.
* Walk 20 min.
* If you hear voices which are not heard by other people, ask yourself if it is possible to ignore them.
Yes
Great! In such a case continue ignoring them.
No
You have to learn to ignore the voices.

This Guide will teach you to ignore the voices. Remember: even if you cannot stop the voices, the voices cannot stop you to live a normal life.

If you believe in things which other people consider strange, try to keep your strange believes for yourself. Everybody has to make the selection of what can be told to other people and what must be private. Believe me, many people have strange believes. Even much stranger than yours. And they are not considered to be sick. Why? Because they keep their strange believes for themselves. That is the secret.

***

Evening

- Think of three different words, any words which just come to your mind at the moment and make a simple story using these 3 words. Repeat 3 times.
- Try to concentrate on an object close to you, any object. What do you feel when looking at the object? What thoughts come to your mind when looking at the object?
- Small supper.

- Nice talk (no complaints) 10 min. When nobody to talk with, phone or internet conversation oral or written.
- Walk 10 min.
- If you hear voices which are not heard by other people, ask yourself if it is possible to ignore them.

Yes

Great! In such a case continue ignoring them.

No

You have to learn to ignore the voices.
This Guide will teach you to ignore the voices.
Remember: even if you cannot stop the voices, the voices cannot stop you to live a normal life.

If you believe in things which other people consider strange, try to keep your strange believes for yourself. Everybody has to make the selection of what can be told to other people and what must be private. Believe me, many people have strange believes. Even much stranger than yours. And they are not considered to be sick. Why? Because they keep their strange believes for themselves. That is the secret.

***

Night

Before sleep
- Take a shower (warm water) 1 min.
- Small physical excercise 3 min.

In Bed
- Repeat STOP (10 times if you hear the voices.
- Think of three different words, any words which just come to your mind at the moment and make a simple story using these 3 words. Repeat untill you fall asleep.

If you cannot fall asleep
- Think of three different words, any words which just come to your mind at the moment and make a simple story using these 3 words. Repeat untill you fall asleep.

If above does not help
- Stand up and go to the toilet (when possible with as little light as possible)
- Think of three different words, any words which just come to your mind at the moment and make a simple story using these 3 words. Repeat untill you fall asleep.

If above does not help
- Say STOP untill you fall asleep

If above does not help
- Go to the kitchen and have a very small snack.

- Back to the bed think of three different words, any words which just come to your mind at the moment and make a simple story using these 3 words. Repeat untill you fall asleep.
- If above does not help think of three different words, any words which just come to your mind at the moment and make a simple story using these 3 words. Repeat untill you fall asleep.

***

Day 5

Morning

* Say STOP when the voices you hear in your head become too loud to hear your own thoughts.
* If above does not help to stop the voices, just turn your attention away from the voices. The best way to turn your attention away from the voices in your head is by doing one of your favorite occupations. Do not be ashamed of any occupation to turn your attention away from the voices in your head. ALWAYS be busy with your favorite occupation when unsupportable voices come to your head.

* Be careful to keep for yourself these of your believes which are found to be strange by the people.
* CONTROL what you say. Say only things which are not strange for the people. You surely already know which of your believes are found to be strange by the people.
* If you do not know yet which of your believes are found to be strange by the people, OBSERVE how people react on what you say. If you see that people are ALERTED by your believes, it means your believes are strange. From now on AVOID presenting such believes.
* Think of three different words, any words which just come to your mind at the moment and make a simple story using these 3 words. Repeat 3 times.
* Try to concentrate on an object close to you, any object. What do you feel when looking at the object? What thoughts come to your mind when looking at the object?
* Small physical excercise (10 min)
* Small breakfast.
* Nice talk (no complaints, no problematic questions) 10 min. When nobody to talk with, phone or internet conversation oral or written.

* Walk 15 min.
* If you hear voices which are not heard by other people, ask yourself if it is possible to ignore the voices.

Yes

Great! In such a case continue ignoring them.

No

You have to learn to ignore the voices.
This Guide will teach you to ignore the voices. Remember: even if you cannot stop the voices, the voices cannot stop you to live a normal life.

If you believe in things which other people consider strange, try to keep your strange believes for yourself. Everybody has to make the selection of what can be told to other people and what must be private. Believe me, many people have strange believes. Even much stranger than yours. And they are not considered to be sick. Why? Because they keep their strange believes for themselves. That is the secret.

***

Afternoon

* Think of three different words, any words which just come to your mind at the moment and make a simple story using these 3 words. Repeat 3 times.
* Try to concentrate on an object close to you, any object. What do you feel when looking at the object? What thoughts come to your mind when looking at the object?
* Dinner and half an hour break (you can sleep).
* Nice talk (no complaints) 15 min. When nobody to talk with, phone or internet conversation oral or written.
* Walk 20 min.
* If you hear voices which are not heard by other people, ask yourself if it is possible to ignore them.

Yes

Great! In such a case continue ignoring them.

No

You have to learn to ignore the voices.
This Guide will teach you to ignore the voices.
Remember: even if you cannot stop the voices, the voices cannot stop you to live a normal life.

If you believe in things which other people consider strange, try to keep your strange

believes for yourself. Everybody has to make the selection of what can be told to other people and what must be private. Believe me, many people have strange believes. Even much stranger than yours. And they are not considered to be sick. Why? Because they keep their strange believes for themselves. That is the secret.

***

Evening

- Think of three different words, any words which just come to your mind at the moment and make a simple story using these 3 words. Repeat 3 times.
- Try to concentrate on an object close to you, any object. What do you feel when looking at the object? What thoughts come to your mind when looking at the object?
- Small supper.
- Nice talk (no complaints) 10 min. When nobody to talk with, phone or internet conversation oral or written.
- Walk 10 min.

- If you hear voices which are not heard by other people, ask yourself if it is possible to ignore them.

Yes

Great! In such a case continue ignoring them.

No

You have to learn to ignore the voices. This Guide will teach you to ignore the voices. Remember: even if you cannot stop the voices, the voices cannot stop you to live a normal life.

If you believe in things which other people consider strange, try to keep your strange believes for yourself. Everybody has to make the selection of what can be told to other people and what must be private. Believe me, many people have strange believes. Even much stranger than yours. And they are not considered to be sick. Why? Because they keep their strange believes for themselves. That is the secret.

***

Night

Before sleep
- Take a shower (warm water) 1 min.
- Small physical excercise 3 min.

In Bed
- Repeat STOP (10 times if you hear the voices.
- Think of three different words, any words which just come to your mind at the moment and make a simple story using these 3 words. Repeat untill you fall asleep.

If you cannot fall asleep
- Think of three different words, any words which just come to your mind at the moment and make a simple story using these 3 words. Repeat untill you fall asleep.

If above does not help
- Stand up and go to the toilet (when possible with as little light as possible)
- Think of three different words, any words which just come to your mind at the moment and make a simple story using these 3 words. Repeat untill you fall asleep.

If above does not help
- Say STOP untill you fall asleep

If above does not help
- Go to the kitchen and have a very small snack.
- Back to the bed think of three different words, any words which just come to your mind at the moment and make a simple story using these 3 words. Repeat untill you fall asleep.

- If above does not help think of three different words, any words which just come to your mind at the moment and make a simple story using these 3 words. Repeat untill you fall asleep.

***

Day 6

Morning

* Say STOP when the voices you hear in your head become too loud to hear your own thoughts.
* If above does not help to stop the voices, just turn your attention away from the voices. The best way to turn your attention away from the voices in your head is by doing one of your favorite occupations. Do not be ashamed of any occupation to turn your attention away from the voices in your head. ALWAYS be busy with your favorite occupation when unsupportable voices come to your head.
* Be careful to keep for yourself these of your believes which are found to be strange by the people.
* CONTROL what you say. Say only things which are not strange for the people. You surely

already know which of your believes are found to be strange by the people.
* If you do not know yet which of your believes are found to be strange by the people, OBSERVE how people react on what you say. If you see that people are ALERTED by your believes, it means your believes are strange. From now on AVOID presenting such believes.
* Think of three different words, any words which just come to your mind at the moment and make a simple story using these 3 words. Repeat 3 times.
* Try to concentrate on an object close to you, any object. What do you feel when looking at the object? What thoughts come to your mind when looking at the object?
* Small physical excercise (10 min)
* Small breakfast.
* Nice talk (no complaints, no problematic questions) 10 min. When nobody to talk with, phone or internet conversation oral or written.
* Walk 15 min.
* If you hear voices which are not heard by other people, ask yourself if it is possible to ignore the voices.
Yes

Great! In such a case continue ignoring them.
No
You have to learn to ignore the voices.
This Guide will teach you to ignore the voices.
Remember: even if you cannot stop the voices, the voices cannot stop you to live a normal life.

If you believe in things which other people consider strange, try to keep your strange believes for yourself. Everybody has to make the selection of what can be told to other people and what must be private. Believe me, many people have strange believes. Even much stranger than yours. And they are not considered to be sick. Why? Because they keep their strange believes for themselves. That is the secret.

***

Afternoon
* Think of three different words, any words which just come to your mind at the moment and make a simple story using these 3 words. Repeat 3 times.
* Try to concentrate on an object close to you, any object. What do you feel when looking at

the object? What thoughts come to your mind when looking at the object?
* Dinner and half an hour break (you can sleep).
* Nice talk (no complaints) 15 min. When nobody to talk with, phone or internet conversation oral or written.
* Walk 20 min.
* If you hear voices which are not heard by other people, ask yourself if it is possible to ignore them.
Yes
Great! In such a case continue ignoring them.
No
You have to learn to ignore the voices.
This Guide will teach you to ignore the voices.
Remember: even if you cannot stop the voices, the voices cannot stop you to live a normal life.

If you believe in things which other people consider strange, try to keep your strange believes for yourself. Everybody has to make the selection of what can be told to other people and what must be private. Believe me, many people have strange believes. Even much stranger than yours. And they are not considered to be sick. Why? Because they keep

their strange believes for themselves. That is the secret.

***

Evening

- Think of three different words, any words which just come to your mind at the moment and make a simple story using these 3 words. Repeat 3 times.
- Try to concentrate on an object close to you, any object. What do you feel when looking at the object? What thoughts come to your mind when looking at the object?
- Small supper.
- Nice talk (no complaints) 10 min. When nobody to talk with, phone or internet conversation oral or written.
- Walk 10 min.
- If you hear voices which are not heard by other people, ask yourself if it is possible to ignore them.

Yes

Great! In such a case continue ignoring them.

No

You have to learn to ignore the voices.

This Guide will teach you to ignore the voices.

Remember: even if you cannot stop the voices, the voices cannot stop you to live a normal life.

If you believe in things which other people consider strange, try to keep your strange believes for yourself. Everybody has to make the selection of what can be told to other people and what must be private. Believe me, many people have strange believes. Even much stranger than yours. And they are not considered to be sick. Why? Because they keep their strange believes for themselves. That is the secret.

***

Night
Before sleep
- Take a shower (warm water) 1 min.
- Small physical excercise 3 min.

In Bed
- Repeat STOP (10 times if you hear the voices.
- Think of three different words, any words which just come to your mind at the moment and make a simple story using these 3 words. Repeat untill you fall asleep.

If you cannot fall asleep

- Think of three different words, any words which just come to your mind at the moment and make a simple story using these 3 words. Repeat untill you fall asleep.

If above does not help
- Stand up and go to the toilet (when possible with as little light as possible)
- Think of three different words, any words which just come to your mind at the moment and make a simple story using these 3 words. Repeat untill you fall asleep.

If above does not help
- Say STOP untill you fall asleep

If above does not help
- Go to the kitchen and have a very small snack.
- Back to the bed think of three different words, any words which just come to your mind at the moment and make a simple story using these 3 words. Repeat untill you fall asleep.
- If above does not help think of three different words, any words which just come to your mind at the moment and make a simple story using these 3 words. Repeat untill you fall asleep.

***

Day 7

Morning
* Say STOP when the voices you hear in your head become too loud to hear your own thoughts.
* If above does not help to stop the voices, just turn your attention away from the voices. The best way to turn your attention away from the voices in your head is by doing one of your favorite occupations. Do not be ashamed of any occupation to turn your attention away from the voices in your head. ALWAYS be busy with your favorite occupation when unsupportable voices come to your head.
* Be careful to keep for yourself these of your believes which are found to be strange by the people.
* CONTROL what you say. Say only things which are not strange for the people. You surely already know which of your believes are found to be strange by the people.
* If you do not know yet which of your believes are found to be strange by the people, OBSERVE how people react on what you say. If you see that people are ALERTED by your believes, it means your believes are strange. From now on AVOID presenting such believes.

* Think of three different words, any words which just come to your mind at the moment and make a simple story using these 3 words. Repeat 3 times.
* Try to concentrate on an object close to you, any object. What do you feel when looking at the object? What thoughts come to your mind when looking at the object?
* Small physical excercise (10 min)
* Small breakfast.
* Nice talk (no complaints, no problematic questions) 10 min. When nobody to talk with, phone or internet conversation oral or written.
* Walk 15 min.
* If you hear voices which are not heard by other people, ask yourself if it is possible to ignore the voices.

Yes

Great! In such a case continue ignoring them.

No

You have to learn to ignore the voices.
This Guide will teach you to ignore the voices.
Remember: even if you cannot stop the voices, the voices cannot stop you to live a normal life.

If you believe in things which other people consider strange, try to keep your strange believes for yourself. Everybody has to make the selection of what can be told to other people and what must be private. Believe me, many people have strange believes. Even much stranger than yours. And they are not considered to be sick. Why? Because they keep their strange believes for themselves. That is the secret.

***

Afternoon
* Think of three different words, any words which just come to your mind at the moment and make a simple story using these 3 words. Repeat 3 times.
* Try to concentrate on an object close to you, any object. What do you feel when looking at the object? What thoughts come to your mind when looking at the object?
* Dinner and half an hour break (you can sleep).
* Nice talk (no complaints) 15 min. When nobody to talk with, phone or internet conversation oral or written.
* Walk 20 min.

* If you hear voices which are not heard by other people, ask yourself if it is possible to ignore them.

Yes

Great! In such a case continue ignoring them.

No

You have to learn to ignore the voices.

This Guide will teach you to ignore the voices. Remember: even if you cannot stop the voices, the voices cannot stop you to live a normal life.

If you believe in things which other people consider strange, try to keep your strange believes for yourself. Everybody has to make the selection of what can be told to other people and what must be private. Believe me, many people have strange believes. Even much stranger than yours. And they are not considered to be sick. Why? Because they keep their strange believes for themselves. That is the secret.

***

Evening

- Think of three different words, any words which just come to your mind at the moment

and make a simple story using these 3 words. Repeat 3 times.
- Try to concentrate on an object close to you, any object. What do you feel when looking at the object? What thoughts come to your mind when looking at the object?
- Small supper.
- Nice talk (no complaints) 10 min. When nobody to talk with, phone or internet conversation oral or written.
- Walk 10 min.
- If you hear voices which are not heard by other people, ask yourself if it is possible to ignore them.

Yes

Great! In such a case continue ignoring them.

No

You have to learn to ignore the voices.
This Guide will teach you to ignore the voices.
Remember: even if you cannot stop the voices, the voices cannot stop you to live a normal life.

If you believe in things which other people consider strange, try to keep your strange believes for yourself. Everybody has to make the selection of what can be told to other people

and what must be private. Believe me, many people have strange believes. Even much stranger than yours. And they are not considered to be sick. Why? Because they keep their strange believes for themselves. That is the secret.

***

Night

Before sleep
- Take a shower (warm water) 1 min.
- Small physical excercise 3 min.

In Bed
- Repeat STOP (10 times if you hear the voices.
- Think of three different words, any words which just come to your mind at the moment and make a simple story using these 3 words. Repeat untill you fall asleep.

If you cannot fall asleep
- Think of three different words, any words which just come to your mind at the moment and make a simple story using these 3 words. Repeat untill you fall asleep.

If above does not help
- Stand up and go to the toilet (when possible with as little light as possible)

- Think of three different words, any words which just come to your mind at the moment and make a simple story using these 3 words. Repeat untill you fall asleep.

If above does not help
- Say STOP untill you fall asleep

If above does not help
- Go to the kitchen and have a very small snack.
- Back to the bed think of three different words, any words which just come to your mind at the moment and make a simple story using these 3 words. Repeat untill you fall asleep.
- If above does not help think of three different words, any words which just come to your mind at the moment and make a simple story using these 3 words. Repeat untill you fall asleep.

***

***

Repeat following the example of the Month One still 2 times.

***

After 3 months you have completed the full Schizophrenia Self Therapy SchST course!

Congratulations to you and to the person accompanying you during 3 months. Now, you are no longer schizophrenic person as one used to call you in an unfair way so far. Now you are a normal person and enjoy it by living a full and happy life!

P. W. Ariveder

www.ingramcontent.com/pod-product-compliance
Lightning Source LLC
Chambersburg PA
CBHW052352220526
45465CB00003BA/1069